Birth
Stories

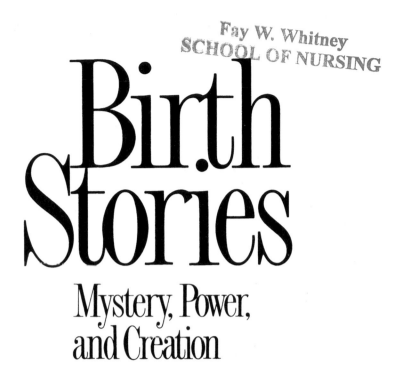

Birth Stories

Mystery, Power, and Creation

Jane Dwinell, R.N.

Bergin & Garvey
Westport, Connecticut • London

Library of Congress Cataloging-in-Publication Data

Dwinell, Jane.
    Birth stories : mystery, power, and creation / Jane Dwinell.
        p.   cm.
    ISBN 0-89789-296-8 (alk. paper). — ISBN 0-89789-304-2 (pbk. :
    alk. paper)
        1. Childbirth—Popular works. 2. Childbirth—Case studies.
    I. Title.
    RG651.D85   1992
    618.4—dc20   92-3348

British Library Cataloguing in Publication Data is available.

Library of Congress Catalog Card Number: 92-3348
ISBN: 0-89789-296-8
        0-89789-304-2 (pbk.)

First published in 1992

Bergin & Garvey, 88 Post Road West, Westport, CT 06881
An imprint of Greenwood Publishing Group, Inc.

Printed in the United States of America

The paper used in this book complies with the
Permanent Paper Standard issued by the National
Information Standards Organization (Z39.48-1984).

10 9 8 7 6

To Sky

Contents

Acknowledgments

This book has been an integral part of my life for many years, ever since a little voice inside me said, "You should go to nursing school and become a midwife." I had had no clear interest in childbirth until then. It was 1975, and I was twenty-two years old. Along the way several people have been important players in my journey, and I would like to thank them.

In nursing school I was fortunate to be guided by Judith. Although her specialty was not obstetrics, she instilled in me the importance of the patient's rights—that it is a nurse's primary duty to speak up for the patient even if it means questioning a doctor's orders. And Karen, wherever you are now, my comrade throughout the highs and lows of nursing school, thanks for being there.

I have been extraordinarily fortunate to work with a unique group of nurses, midwives, and doctors who believe in the strength of women and the rights of childbearing families. Special thanks to Lou for teaching me so much, and to Nancy and Tina for sharing yourselves and putting up with all my ups and downs.

Thanks to all the families who have allowed me to attend your labors and births—without you this book could not have been written.

I have several women friends who share my love for women and their power, and have supported and encouraged me in many ways: Thanks to Mary, Julie, Polly, Nene, Meg, Val, Cindy, and Catherine for your friendship.

Thanks to my mother for giving birth to me; to my father for telling me I could be whatever I wanted to be; to my brother Bandy for his quiet, steadfast caring; and to my brother James for encouraging my writing and being there during all my various life crises.

To Nancy Cohen, who thought this book was important and put me in touch with Sophy Craze, my thanks to you both.

To the patient and caring birth attendants who helped my children come into this world: thanks to Katra, Kit, Bunny, Laura, Thurmond, Becky, Nancy, and June (what a crowd!) for helping with Dana, and to Claudia and Patty for helping with Sayer.

Most important, my deepest loving thanks to my beloved and best friend, Sky, who has believed in me every step of the way, who read and commented on the entire manuscript, who took care of the homestead and the children while I wrote at all hours of the day and night, who held my hand as I gave birth to our daughter, Dana, and into whose hands our son, Sayer, was born. And to Dana and Sayer, thanks for joining us!

The following stories are based on births I have attended over the years. Names and other identifying information have been changed to protect the privacy of the families involved.

1

Women, Birth, and Power

I love women. I have great respect for their strength and their power. Women are special for many reasons but especially for their ability to conceive, to nurture a new life, and to give birth. Their inner strength and power come from a journey of centuries, as each woman holds in herself the knowledge of her ancestors and all the women who have come before.

Women can conceive, nurture, and give birth to many things besides children. All women, not just those who have given birth to children, need to be respected for that great ability. In today's highly technical reproductive world there seems to be an increased importance being placed on women becoming biological mothers. Women have many new creations to share with the world; their importance should not be based on whether they are biological mothers. Many women have given birth to businesses, buildings, and books, to movies, sculptures, and quilts. There are countless new ideas and inventions that are part of our lives because of women. We should be thankful for so many women who have listened to their inner guidance and nurtured a special idea and worked so hard to breathe life into it.

Although this book is about childbirth, the philosophy is the same whether the birth produces a baby or a business. As women open up to their inner voice, their inner strength, their inner wisdom, they will find they have the power to give birth to anything. The importance of learning to tap into that wisdom and to respect its place and power in the lives of all women is what I want to convey to you.

I believe in the midwifery model of childbirth, not the medical model. Traditional medical practices have lost sight of who is actually giving birth: the pregnant woman. Too often the doctor takes over and controls the pregnancy and delivery. A woman rarely has a chance to speak for herself but is told what she must or must not do, what tests will be performed, and just how many hours she will be allowed to labor before the doctor intervenes to make himself more comfortable.

The midwifery model holds that birth is a woman-centered activity, that it is gentle and peaceful, and comes about at its own speed. A woman is respected, her questions and ideas are respected, and she gives birth when, where, and how she chooses. A midwife is there to guide her, to answer questions, to listen to fears and concerns, to offer different solutions to problems—which may include mainstream medical technology or the use of herbs, visualization, massage, counseling, and caring.

Appropriate technology can be lifesaving and clearly has opened the doors for many more women to give birth. Ultrasound, cesarean sections under spinal anesthesia, genetic testing, blood transfusions, fetal monitors, and neonatal intensive care nurseries have all contributed to saving the lives of women and babies, and have their place in certain situations. *But* these same technologies have cost consumers incredible amounts of money in increased health insurance costs, doctor's office costs, hospital costs, and medical malpractice costs because these technologies have been used excessively, routinely, instead of as special, rarely used, lifesaving procedures. Doctors are now expected to produce perfect babies. The malpractice arena has scared doctors into practicing defensive medicine or getting out of obstetrics altogether.

There is an answer here, and the pregnant woman holds the key. By choosing a midwife (or one of the rare physicians who do practice the midwifery model), by taking responsibility for herself and her child, by saying "no" to certain technologies, by finding solutions that are not so intrusive and expensive, by educating herself about her health and her choices, a woman can turn things around. Instead of being pregnant and giving birth in a fear-based mode, a woman can use the time to look inside herself, to learn about the power she holds, the wisdom that she knows, to trust herself and her instincts, and then to give birth with that sense of clarity and honesty.

Being pregnant is not 100 percent comfortable, and giving birth is not painless. Doctors, childbirth educators, and nurses who promise this are taking power from the woman and setting her up in a system of dishonesty. If a woman thinks that by following a certain breathing pattern her labor will be painless, she will become quite distressed when she discovers otherwise, and will often blame herself for her "failure." If the blame she places on herself doesn't increase the pain of her contractions and slow down the process, then the doctor's or nurse's suggestion that she have some pain medication will. The woman will then give her power over to her attendants, who will place her on the medical merry-go-round (which they prefer because it is organized and planned and gives them something to do).

Here's a typical merry-go-round scenario:

A woman arrives at a hospital in labor. She is interviewed for admission, has blood drawn, and gives a urine sample. She is told to change into a hospital "johnny," a very uncomfortable piece of clothing. She is required to lie in bed attached to a fetal monitor for a "twenty minute strip" to make sure the baby's "OK." She is denied food and drink. Her partner may or may not be present during these activities. When they are over, no one suggests that she move around or do something to make herself more comfortable and at ease. Meanwhile, her labor continues.

She stays in bed either because the nurse has left on the fetal monitor (for convenience, safety, hospital policy, or some other lame excuse) or because the woman is afraid of doing something "wrong" or speaking up for herself. The contractions begin to hurt more with her anxiety, her position, and the progression of labor. She may begin to moan, cry, or make more noise than previously. Instead of speaking to the woman's strength and encouraging a change of position, the nurse, trying to comfort her, suggests some pain medication to "make the pain go away" or "take the edge off."

The woman, scared and feeling like a failure, takes the medication. The medication makes her groggy and, eventually, more uncomfortable. The nurse offers her more. The woman sleeps between contractions and wakes up petrified and frantic as each contraction begins. She has probably been hooked up to the fetal monitor again. The medication, her position, and her anxiety have slowed the contractions, so she is no longer dilating according to the "curve." The hospital staff starts administrating Pitocin to speed up the contractions. She starts screaming and gets "out of control" because the induced contractions hurt more. More pain medication is given. Her bag of waters is broken and countless vaginal exams are done. Because the woman is scared, lying on her back, and full of drugs, the baby begins to show signs of stress. The doctor, fed up with the slowness of the process and afraid of a lawsuit if the baby has a problem, suggests a cesarean. The woman, so scared, so fuzzy, and in so much pain, says, "Yes, doctor, please make the pain go away. Thank you, thank you, doctor, for delivering my baby and making the pain go away."

Because the mother has had surgery (cesarean or episiotomy) and is groggy from the drugs, her baby is taken to the nursery. There it is weighed, measured, bathed, diapered, and placed in a bright, soundless, motionless isolette, whereupon it is ignored except for having its vital signs taken every few minutes. Perhaps it is taken to the mother for a short visit or given to the father for a brief hold. It lives in the nursery for the next several days, seeing its mother only for brief periods every few hours for feedings. After a few days, mother and baby, strangers to one another, go home. The mother, exhausted, scared, and helpless, finds it very hard to provide for the needs of her newborn.

This scenario is repeated day after day in hospitals across this country. Cesarean rates are commonly 25 to 30 percent in most hospitals. If a woman does not have a cesarean, she may have an epidural with a forceps or suction delivery. (And people wonder why the cost of medical care is high.)

Contrast the merry-go-round with this woman-centered scenario:

A woman is in labor. She is in her own clothing or naked, however she is comfortable. She may be at home or at a birthing center. Her partner and other support people of her choice are with her. She is free to do as she wishes—walk around, lie down, eat, drink, shower, dance, sing, laugh, or scream. Unobtrusively, the midwife or nurse periodically listens to the baby's heartbeat with a fetoscope or Doptone. Those in attendance are patient, loving, quiet, and respectful. They may offer suggestions, rub the woman's back, hand her wet washcloths and cold drinks. Time is endless and time is now. There is no rush.

Labor progresses, and everyone works together, supporting each other. The woman is central and strong. She may be angry, happy, frustrated, in pain, or tired. Her attendants speak to her strength and power. They do what they can to help her find that place which will help her go on.

Eventually, she becomes fully dilated and begins to push. She may be squatting or lying down, she may be sitting or standing, she may be indoors or outside. Slowly the baby's head and body emerge into someone's hands— the woman's, the midwife's, the partner's—and is laid upon the mother's belly. Baby and mother are covered with warm blankets. The baby nurses when it is ready, and the new family gets acquainted. The birth attendants carefully but unobtrusively watch the woman and baby for any postbirth problems. When they are assured all is well, the family is left alone to rest and snuggle and talk to friends and relatives.

For the next several days the parents, the new baby, and any siblings are together, enjoying each other's presence and getting to know each other. The midwife or nurse checks in periodically to answer questions and to make sure everyone is doing well. They eat food that they like, they sleep in a comfortable bed, and they begin the hard work of parenting a new being. In contrast with the exhausted woman just off the merry-go-round, they have the strength and power that come with a woman-centered birth to help them on their way.

I say it's time to stop the merry-go-round and give birth back to women. Even if a woman is not aware of any of her power and wisdom during pregnancy, an aware and respectful birth attendant can help her tap into that power and guide her to give birth to her child. The woman will emerge from her experience with a sense of self-worth and empowerment that will carry her into the rest of her life. Motherhood will be easier, and any other endeavor she chooses will also be easier. She will know deep inside of her that she gave birth to her own child under her own steam, and if she can do that, she can do anything!

I present to you my philosophy of childbirth. I do not pretend that this is a how-to book or one full of medical information. It is the story of my journey as a childbirth attendant: as a nurse in a medical center, in an in-hospital birthing center, and at home. It is the story of the wisdom I have gained and that I want to share with you: the pregnant woman, her partner and friends, obstetric nurses, midwives, childbirth educators, and physicians who care. I have attended several thousand labors and births, and will share some of those experiences, in my words and from my perspective. I will share some labors and births that illustrate my philosophy that all women are different, all babies are different, all labors are different, and that birth attendants must respect those differences, learn from them, and trust them. One day I hope to see a society where all women and children are respected for who they are and what they have to offer, and that woman-centered childbirth will be the primal starting point.

2

Kitty

Ruptured Membranes

Kitty arrived at the birthing center with her partner, Chuck. She was expecting her first baby, and she was thirty-seven weeks pregnant. Her water had broken the day before. She and Chuck had waited for the beginning of labor, had walked around their mountain home, and had made love without vaginal penetration. No contractions, no labor. Only the endless drip, drip, drip of clear amniotic fluid. They came to the birthing center to wait and to have Kitty's blood and temperature checked periodically for signs of infection.

They settled into a room and relaxed together. They read and napped and took more long walks. All tests continued to check out fine—no signs of infection. They watched several women come to the center, give birth, and go home with their newborns. I could see the jealousy and want in Kitty's eyes. She, too, wanted a baby to hold in her arms.

I was working the night shift three days after Kitty and Chuck came to the hospital. We had been busy with a birth and had not been in to see them; best to let them sleep. We would listen for the next time Kitty used the bathroom to check her temperature and the baby's heartbeat.

About 3:30 A.M. Kitty came out of her room and started walking up and down the hall. I went over to talk with her, and she said she didn't feel well, thought she was coming down with something. She'd been having diarrhea, couldn't sleep, and felt a bit nauseated, too. She had come out into the hallway because she didn't want to wake Chuck. I checked her temperature and the heartbeat—all was fine. I offered her some ginger ale, which she accepted gladly and drank heartily.

Kitty said she felt a little better but was going to keep walking around. I went back to the nurses' station. I heard her go back in her room to use the toilet. About ten minutes later she came out of the room and started pacing the hall again. When I asked her how she was feeling, she said, "Much worse."

It suddenly dawned on me that Kitty might be in labor, so I started walking with her. Sure enough, about every two minutes she rubbed her belly for forty-five seconds or so, then stopped. She said she was having terrible cramps but didn't have diarrhea anymore. I asked if I could feel her belly the next time a "cramp" came and told her I suspected that she might be in labor.

"Really? No wonder I feel so weird."

After feeling several strong contractions, listening to the baby again, and confirming that she was truly in labor, I asked if I could do a vaginal exam.

We went back to their room, and Chuck slept through it all. Kitty was a very stretchy eight centimeters. I told her I was going to call her midwife, and Kitty leaned over to wake up Chuck.

I left the room, told the other nurse on duty what was happening, called the midwife, and gathered the birthing supplies. By the time I got back to the room, Kitty was holding onto Chuck, moaning softly, and saying that she thought she had to push. Another contraction came, and involuntarily she let out a low groan and pushed at the peak of the contraction. The midwife opened the door.

"Somebody having a baby in here?" she said with a smile. Kitty fell into her arms, laughing and crying.

Kitty squatted and pushed with the next contraction, holding onto the end of the bed. She did that for a couple more contractions, then moved to the bed, where she got into a semi-reclining position, grabbed her knees, and pushed again. Her perineum bulged, and we could see wisps of hair. Chuck had her nestled in his arms as she pushed again, slowly and steadily. The baby's head emerged, then the shoulders, and finally the entire baby slithered out into the midwife's hands.

"It's a boy!" she said as she laid Luke on Kitty's belly. Chuck and Kitty and Luke were all crying; the midwife and I just smiled. Luke was small but well-built. I dried him off and covered the new family with warm blankets—Chuck had removed his shirt and crawled under the covers. A few minutes later the placenta came and Kitty's perineum was checked—no tears. It was not quite 5 A.M.

I tidied up, and the midwife went home to get a bit more sleep. Luke nursed well and then was held by his father while Kitty got up and showered. While I was in the bathroom helping her, she mused on her labor.

"That wasn't anything like I expected. I really thought I was just getting the flu. I mean, it hurt, but not that bad. Well, and then when I found out I was in labor, I was just so excited I hardly felt a thing!" Kitty was glowing with the typical postbirth high.

Kitty, Chuck, and Luke ended up staying another four days—Luke was jaundiced due to his small size and slight prematurity—and had to spend some time under the lights. When he wasn't nursing, he slept in an isolette with special lights shining on his bare skin. The lights helped to break down the excess bilirubin that had accumulated in his blood and turned his skin yellow. He seemed happy to bask in the warmth and equally happy to lie nestled at his mother's breast. When his bilirubin had dropped to a safe level, the family went home—a little more than a week after they came. It was unusual to have a family with us for so long, and we were sorry to see them leave. But we were happy that things had turned out so well, jaundice notwithstanding: that Kitty's labor had started spontaneously, and that Luke showed no effects from the early loss of his protected watery home.

*   *   *

Rupture of the membranes. Breaking of the waters. Something that has to happen before a baby is born into the fresh air of life. Rarely is a baby born in the caul—with the membranes intact—a spectacular sight. The baby emerges as if in a space suit; the face and head are surrounded by a watery bubble. The birth attendant must then rip the covering so that the baby can breathe. A beautiful but very wet event!

More often than not, the waters break before birth, usually during labor. Sometimes they break before labor begins—and sometimes labor does not begin for several days. Most doctors believe in the old adage that a baby must be born within eighteen to twenty-four hours after the break because of the possibility of infection. But a study done at a major medical center showed this to not be necessarily true—that a woman can be watched, her blood tested daily, and her temperature, pulse, and the baby's heartbeat checked every four hours. A change in any of these can indicate infection and the necessity to induce labor to get the baby born—otherwise there is no need to interfere.

There are several issues here. One is breaking the waters—when, how, and why. The other is what to do after they have broken.

Most doctors break the waters at some point in labor if they have not broken before. They have several reasons for doing this. One, they think it may stimulate the labor to go faster. Two, they can see the color of the fluid to know if there is any meconium staining. Three, they like to have something to do and to have something for the nurses to do (clean up!). Four, it commits them to getting the baby out within a certain time frame; doctors rarely have the patience to let nature take her course. Most doctors break the waters without discussing it with the woman and her partner, and sometimes without even warning the nurse, who generally likes to prepare for the mess and listen to the baby's heartbeat at the same time.

None of these are valid reasons. Although I have seen labors that seemed to be stimulated after the waters were broken, there were plenty of other times when it did nothing. Many midwives claim it slows things or makes the contractions more painful to the woman's perception even though the increased strength is not dilating the cervix any faster.

As with any labor- and birth-related procedure, breaking the waters needs to be discussed before it is done. It certainly can be done as another step toward increasing the strength of a slowing labor—after breast stimulation and walking and before Pitocin—with the knowledge that, like the other options, it may or may not work. It can be useful to check to the color of the fluid as the woman nears full dilation at a home birth, to prepare for a hospital transfer if there is much meconium. That observation is unnecessary in a hospital because all resuscitation and suctioning equipment is readied before every birth.

As for premature or prolonged rupture of the membranes—that is, before labor begins, with no contractions by twelve to twenty-four hours later—there is no need for routine Pitocin induction. If a woman is near term, she can attempt to stimulate labor with activity, herbs, castor oil, orgasms, or breast stimulation. (If she is before thirty-six or thirty-seven weeks, it is best to let the baby stay inside a bit longer anyway.) Pitocin should be started only when signs of infection are present—as in the story of Laura,

Mark, and Catherine in Chapter 7. Once we clearly insti-
tuted the "wait and watch" policy at the birthing center, it
was obvious that most women went into labor within
three days. Although a few women began to show signs of
infection and were induced, Catherine was the only baby
to be seriously affected during my five years at the center.

Why are so many institutions unable or unwilling to
trust this policy? Is it the fear of malpractice suits in case of
a sick baby? Is it habit? Is it the doctor's impatience with
the mystery and the spontaneity of labor? Is it the inability
to trust, to sit back, and to let the woman do the work?
Probably it is a combination of all of these. It is up to the
woman to discuss this issue with her birth attendant—
both what to do if the waters break and labor does not begin right away, and what to do if the waters do not break
during labor. I have seen doctors happy to abide by a
woman's wish not to have her waters broken—*if she speaks
up prior to labor.* Otherwise, the same doctors will routinely
break them at some point, usually around eight centimeters.

The amniotic sac and the warm water it contains are a
home and safe playground for the baby. A place where the
baby floats and stretches and experiments with its mus-
cles. A cushion against the bumps and jolts of the
mother's daily life. A fluid the baby drinks and pees, testing its digestive tract absorption, its kidneys, and its bladder. A protection from the normal and abnormal bacteria
of the birth canal. Continually made and processed, amniotic fluid never dries up. It surrounds the baby or it runs
out of the woman's vagina—a wet omen of the birth to
come. When the amniotic sac breaks on its own, it signals
another mystery of the birth process. When it is broken by
a routine-loving doctor, it is another interference with a
natural process, a sign that the doctor does not trust.
Which would you rather have?

3

Cindy

An "Accidental" Natural Birth

On a clear, bright Saturday morning, I was on duty with one other nurse. The birthing center was quiet—just a couple of women and their babies getting ready to go home. We were having a cup of tea while the women ate breakfast, talking about canning and fall gardening. The phone rang; it was the woman from the admissions desk.

"There's a woman down here that thinks she's in labor."

"What's her name?" I asked, checking our "due list."

"Cindy Rivers. She says she's not from around here."

"Send her up," I said. "We'll talk to her and see what's going on."

A few minutes later a man and a woman walked down the hall, looking nervous. Cindy was quite pregnant—close to term, by my guess. I directed them to the nearest vacant room.

Cindy and Mason Rivers were vacationing; she was thirty-six weeks pregnant and her doctor had O.K.'d this last out-of-state trip. Cindy and Mason were looking for land and wanted to move to the area. Her waters had broken that morning at the motel, and this was the closest hospital. Cindy was having mild contractions every seven or eight minutes.

"You've got to call my doctor right away," she said. "I'm very high risk, and I need special medication and special facilities for the delivery."

She was so nervous and scared that I took down the information. I explained that I would need to get one of our doctors to see her and have him contact her doctor. I told her about the birthing center—that we generally did not handle complicated pregnancies and that all babies were born in the birthing rooms. I asked her what made her high risk.

"My age! I'm nearly forty, and we tried for years to get pregnant. Plus I have asthma, and the doctor said that would be dangerous when I was in labor. I am in labor, right?"

I assured her that she was in labor but that it was still early. I also did not think that asthma was that great a complication—nor was age—to necessitate a high-risk birth.

"Oh, I really wanted to have a natural birth and my baby in a birthing room and everything, but the doctor said no, it was absolutely too dangerous. Are you sure it's OK?"

I told her I thought so, but in any case, she didn't have too many other options. I called one of the doctors.

By the time he arrived, Cindy's contractions had gotten closer together, longer, and stronger. I had spoken with Cindy's out-of-state doctor, had taken down the list of asthma medications she would need—intravenously—and showed the list to our doctor.

"Heavens, she doesn't need all that," was his reply.

Cindy and Mason were relaxing on the bed when the doctor and I came into the room. He introduced himself and began talking with them about Cindy's labor and her pregnancy history. Cindy's labor was growing in intensity, and the doctor asked if he could do a vaginal exam.

Cindy was excited to find out how far dilated she was, and even more excited when the doctor reported eight centimeters.

"But what about my special medications and a delivery room and everything?" Cindy asked.

"You don't need all that," explained the doctor. "Things are moving right along, you're doing fine. If you stay relaxed and keep moving with your labor, you won't need any medicine. You just let us know if you're having any trouble breathing and we'll help. Otherwise, I say it's best to let things alone. You're having a baby, and that's not a problem." He smiled and left the room.

Cindy and Mason were both excited and concerned. It had been drilled into them for so many months that Cindy could not have a natural birth because of her age and her asthma. In a few minutes, not only were they having their baby away from home, but they had been told her "high risk" label was irrelevant. They didn't have much time to brood on it because Cindy's labor demanded their attention.

The other nurse and I stayed with Cindy and Mason. They had not attended childbirth classes, because their doctor had said it was not important. We did our best to explain what was happening and what would be happening, and to help them with the contractions, which were getting more intense. Cindy leaned on Mason as the other nurse pressed her lower back, and I spoke quietly to her, encouraging her to relax. The baby's heartbeat was fine, and Cindy was not having any trouble breathing, even with the added stress of the unknown.

After about forty-five minutes, the doctor reappeared just as Cindy began feeling pressure. She climbed up on the bed, where a vaginal exam confirmed she was fully dilated. The doctor did some perineal massage as Cindy began to push. He helped her stretch gently as she bore down. I readied the equipment for the birth. Slowly, slowly, with each push her perineum bulged more and more until at last we could see the wrinkled head making its way out. Cindy gave one long, low push, and the baby's head slipped out. I encouraged her to reach down and touch the baby's head as she gave another push for the shoulders, and the baby slipped out.

The baby was small but breathed right away and pinked up quickly. We dried her off as she lay on Cindy's belly. Cindy and Mason were crying and saying over and over, "I don't believe it, I don't believe it, we got to have the baby right here."

Heather looked at her parents, blinking in the bright light of that fall morning. It was barely two hours after Cindy and Mason had arrived. The doctor shook their hands and said "Good job" as he left the room. The other nurse helped Heather get on the breast while I cleaned up, then we both left the room.

Cindy, Mason, and Heather stayed with us for a week. Heather, a sturdy and strong five and half pounds, became jaundiced and had to spend some time under the lights. While Heather was "sunbathing," I had many conversations with Cindy about her labor and birth, trying to help her understand why her doctor had said one thing, and then something completely different had happened. I mostly listened as she talked of her confusion, her sense of betrayal by her doctor, and her delight at having her baby the way she had dreamed. I wondered about all the other women under this doctor's care, and others like him, who were not being allowed, to have the kind of birth that they wanted. I was as delighted as Cindy that they had happened by and shared their birth with us—an important experience for everyone.

* * *

What happened here? Were we wrong not to follow doctor's orders? Or were we right to take a wait-and-see attitude and let Cindy do what she wanted? Things turned out fine—Cindy had no breathing problems during labor or anytime during their stay. What was the city doctor's real concern—that he produce a healthy baby for Cindy and Mason, something they had wanted for a long time? Or was he truly worried about Cindy's age and asthma?

Age meant nothing to me. I had seen women from fourteen to forty-four give birth. Other than individual differences in attitude, knowledge, and body tone, there never seemed to be anything particularly notable about an older woman giving birth. Some were athletes having their first baby, others were housewives having their fifth or sixth, still others were women in their second marriage having a "love child" with support from their teenage children from the first marriage. There were as many different circumstances as women.

The babies were no different either. Although babies of older mothers can have more genetic problems, those problems are usually long-resolved during pregnancy and have no direct bearing on the birth. I certainly could never tell the difference between a baby of a teen mother and a forty-year-old mother. They are all babies with the same wants and needs—food, warmth, cuddling, and dry diapers.

I learned about the real world from Cindy, about the attitude of doctors who want to be in control of a labor and birth ("delivery" to them), doctors who put the wants and needs of the woman—the "vessel"—secondary to the doctor's comfort and feelings of safety and perfection. I was used to a small group of doctors and midwives who let nature take her course, ever vigilant for problems that would need intervention but otherwise staying out of it. It was frightening to be reminded that doctors like Cindy's exist, and are, in fact, the norm.

I had watched Cindy over the week and listened to her while she expressed her feelings of anger, betrayal, and, finally, joy and strength. She had always been afraid of her body, for years relying on doctors to help her—first with her asthma and then with her infertility. She had turned herself over to them, and the reality of having her own strength shocked her. Because so much of the medical care in this country is based on ill-ness instead of well-ness, Cindy had never been encouraged to do her own healing, to educate herself about her body, and to discover why she had trouble breathing or trouble conceiving. She had relied on doctors to tell her what was wrong and to "fix" it with pills and surgery.

Now she was beginning to trust her body, to trust her self, to decide what was best for her. I watched her questioning the doctors about Heather's jaundice. She seemed to take nothing for granted anymore. She had questions and she wanted answers, she wanted to trust. She was becoming empowered and beginning to believe in her own strength as a woman and a mother.

How many other women out there are being steamrollered every day by their doctors, believing that only the doctor holds the answers to their problems, that only the doctor can make everything better? How does that feeling of helplessness transfer to other parts of their lives? They may feel too helpless to work on changing a bad marriage or to leave the relationship altogether. They may want their partner to take a more active role in parenting and housework. They may be unable to deal with an abusive childhood or a dead-end job or a dying parent. They may feel that their problems need to be handled by others— professionals with "magic" answers and treatments.

Certainly there are physical and mental health problems that require help from others to be healed. A compatible therapist or support group may be necessary to begin the healing of a broken childhood. Hormones or surgery may be necessary to help an infertile woman conceive. Career counseling or a stay at a battered women's shelter may help a woman move on to a better life. But mainly, the best help, the most long-lasting healing, needs to come from within. The most advanced technologies may change our bodies, but only we can change our minds, our attitudes toward health, healing, and the power and strength of each individual body to know what is best.

Cindy's story clearly illustrates that fact—she was able to give birth herself, without high-tech intrusions. She only needed to be given the space and support and knowledge that she could do it herself. We simply stood by and watched. Cindy did all of the work. I would hope for the same for all pregnant women—knowledge, respect, and space to do what their body already knows how to do so beautifully.

4

Susan

Birth/Death

I'll never forget the bright February Friday afternoon when I was told of an impending birth and death. Susan and Larry were expecting their second child. Susan was planning a vaginal birth after her previous cesarean (VBAC) and was looking forward to the challenge of birthing her child without surgery. But something wasn't right at the prenatal visit, and they were sent for an ultrasound. Anencephalic. A baby with no brain. Their child, happily kicking and flipping around in utero, heart beating steadily, could not live outside of that special environment. A cesarean was scheduled for Monday. I was the nurse on duty.

I had been helping babies get born for several years; it was my passion and joy. The power of the contractions, the long hours, the emotional outbursts all culminating in one long, slow orgasm, the birth of a child. I had seen twins and two-pound preemies, healthy babies and babies with heart defects, fourteen-pound bruisers and babies with the intestines on the outside of the body. But I had never seen a baby die. Many had come close, but with the precision teamwork of nurses and doctors they had triumphed and survived.

Now I was to assist with a birth and a death. Anencephalic babies can live up to three days, even a week, depending on how little or how much brain they do have. But no one wants them to—it's a struggle for survival that cannot happen, yet no one wants to deny them clean diapers or a nipple to suck on. We would wait and watch and not resuscitate.

Susan and Larry had prepared themselves. They shared their plans with me. They wanted to see the baby, but could I be sure to cover up its head? They wanted time and space to be with their baby and to hold it until it died. They wanted pictures and fingerprints and clothes. They had names picked out and a funeral planned.

Surgery began. It was a familiar team—surgeon and assistant, anesthesiologist, operating room (OR) nurses, family doctor, father, pediatrician, myself—all surrounding the woman carefully draped with only her head exposed. Usually the atmosphere was festive, a baby about to be born; sometimes it was tense if there was fetal distress or a long, hard labor. But nothing was like this: quiet, no one's eyes meeting over their masks.

And then the baby was born. It was a girl, Cecilia. The pediatrician received her into a blanket and carried her over to me. We watched Cecelia blink her eyes and gasp for breath, once, twice. She was warm but blue, and her heart was beating strong. I longed to reach for her, to stimulate her, to help her breathe, as I did so automatically every day, whispering soothing words to a newborn, encouraging him or her to join the world. I held my hands behind my back; I did not touch Cecelia, and I did not speak to her.

I looked at her perfect toes and fingers, all there. Her chubby little legs and arms, her strong torso, her mouth, her nose, her eyes and ears, and then . . . nothing. A grotesque yet strangely cute look, no brain, no forehead, no hair, a slanted line of empty space from eyes to ears to nape of neck. No signals to help her breathe, to tell her to swallow or cry or smile. She blinked her eyes again and tried no more.

I wrapped her carefully and handed her to Larry. I stood and sobbed as I watched Larry and Susan stroke Cecelia and talk to her, explore her body until they were ready to uncover the top of her head. It seemed too private. I turned away and gathered up my equipment, watched the surgery, stared at the walls, anything to stop crying and not intrude.

Susan was getting uncomfortable and was being medicated by the anesthesiologist; she asked Larry to leave and take Cecilia to the nursery. Larry held Cecilia as I walked them down the hall. The pediatrician did a perfunctory exam for the record and left me with the instructions "Check her heartbeat every five minutes and let me know when you don't hear it anymore." Cecelia, blue, getting cold, and brainless, still had a heart that was beating.

I bathed Cecelia, not worrying about chilling her but keeping her warm and comfortable out of habit. I measured and weighed her, placed footprints on a piece of paper, and gave her to Larry to dress. He held her and I took pictures, and then I held her and he took pictures. All the while I was weeping, a steady stream of tears coming out of my eyes. The elderly nursery aide, who had seen babies of all kinds over her forty years of duty, asked me if I wanted her to take over.

"No," I said, "I have to do it myself." I knew I had to deal with this birth/death by experiencing it all.

I put a stethoscope to Cecilia's chest. Her heart was still beating, very faint and slow, forty-five minutes after her birth. Larry carried her to Susan's room, and I left the family alone together. Five minutes later I went in and listened, and there was no heartbeat. I left the room.

Ten minutes later Larry asked me to come in. Cecelia was in bed with Susan, snuggled under the covers, close to her mother's breast, as I had seen so many newborns. Only Cecelia was a deep purple blue, her skin was getting shiny, and she was stiff. I took Cecelia in my arms, her parents said a final good-bye, and I left the room.

My next job was an unpleasant one—to bag and tag Cecelia. In the morgue I took off her little outfit, placed her in a plastic bag, and wrote her name on the cards I tied around her ankle and wrist. That afternoon I would come back to the morgue with professional curiosity and watch Cecelia's autopsy—a perfect baby in every other regard.

I went home and wept for the rest of the day. It was so unfair of whatever God there is to create such a being; it was all part of a cosmic plan; it made me feel lonely and vulnerable. It was so hard not to work to save her life, as I had done over and over again.

I continued to help many babies come into this world after Cecelia's birth and death. I watched them all open their eyes and breathe and cry lustily. In another place I stood by the side of several old people as they struggled to take their last breaths, drowning in their own bodily fluids, and then peacefully breathing no more. But none ever affected me the way Cecelia did. To have birth and death so close together, so intertwined, echoing each other's intensity.

*   *   *

Most childbirth culminates in a happy time with the addition of a new member of a family, challenging the parents to take on a new role and responsibility. Periodically, this does not happen. A baby is stillborn, premature and not expected to live, or severely deformed with no chance of life. A rare and shocking time both for the parents and for the persons in attendance.

Cecelia was the only baby to die in my presence, but I helped several women give birth to their already dead babies and also helped seemingly healthy babies get born, only to have them die, within months, of sudden infant death syndrome (SIDS) or some unexpected illness or accident. I have seen several kinds of deformities, those which can be mended with time and surgery and those which cannot.

We like to have things perfect in this society. People are not comfortable with death, deformity, or various kinds of dis-abilities. We want things whole, "fixed," and "normal," anything to help *us* feel comfortable. Death and disability have been removed from family life with the increase of hospitals and institutions as places to house the dying and different. A century ago people died at home, and handicapped children were cared for by their families. "Flawed" people were a fact of life.

Today there is technology to (theoretically) allow only "perfect" babies to be born into this world. Amniocentesis and other genetic tests, fetal monitoring, stress tests, sophisticated blood tests, ultrasound, and cesarean sections are all supposed to provide perfect babies. But nothing is certain in the world of childbirth. No one can predict when labor will start, when it will end, and what will happen to mother and child at that time. People are only fooling themselves if they think they can produce a perfect baby by choosing the right tests, the right hospital, the right doctor, the right childbirth classes, the right wallpaper in the birthing room.

Babies are born when they are ready to be born, in the way they want/need to be born. This may seem to be an esoteric or radical idea, depending on your personal religious and world views. Some mothers can try to control the birthing process mentally or physically with different drugs and technology, but the great mystery of it all is that no one knows why labor starts and why it takes the amount of time it does, or why it produces a certain outcome. Some things can be controlled, but these are superficial compared with the ultimate, bigger picture.

Laboring women need to give up control to be able to give birth to their children. This may be a contradiction to many childbirth educators who teach weeks of tips and tasks to keep a woman "in control" and breathing "properly." Women will tell you of the feeling of "otherworldliness" just prior to giving birth: "I didn't know where I was." "Everyone seemed so far away." "I don't remember what happened, all I know was that I had to do it." Control relinquished but power remaining, a woman gives birth.

What if she gives birth to a dead or dying child? All I can suggest is that she try to respect that fact and participate as much as possible. Hold that child and touch that child. Be together as a family. Speak to that child. Cry. Rejoice. Let things happen. Don't let the attendants around you interfere with what you need to do as a family. Footprints, measurements, weights, and examinations can wait. The baby belongs with the family, and only the family has the right to say what will happen next.

Perhaps you want all heroic measures taken, perhaps you don't. If you are so fortunate as to have the time to prepare for your baby's death, as Larry and Susan did, you can decide what you would like to do and let those around you know how they can assist you with your plans.

Every pregnant woman worries about the death or deformity of her unborn child at some point during her pregnancy. Her partner may worry, too. Speak about it, bring the worries into the light, and know that they are normal. Like any worries, try not to dwell on them, but accept their existence and know that you have the strength to give birth to your child and accept him or her for who he or she is. That is not an easy task in light of our society's treatment of "imperfect" people, but one that needs to happen. The more we can accept disabled people and death, the healthier our world will be.

5

Shelley

A Three-Generation Birth

It was Christmas. I loved working on the holidays, a birth seemed extra special. It was quiet this Christmas, only one woman in labor. Shelley was twenty-three years old and single. She lived out of state and had returned to her childhood home to give birth to her first child. She wanted assistance from her mother and grandmother.

Shelley was a modern woman—she had moved from the country to the city to have a career and a new life. Her mother, Louise, was a poor country woman, fortyish, factory worker, and mother of four. Grandma, probably in her early sixties, fairly young to be becoming a great-grandmother, was quite a local character, full of life and wit, and a mother of eight.

Shelley was in active labor when she arrived about 9 A.M., and was five to six centimeters dilated. She relaxed in her room, took a shower, and had some toast and juice. I talked with Louise and Grandma and explained what would be happening. The birthing room was still a new concept for the community, and I liked to prepare those who might not understand. It was then I learned their fascinating history.

Louise had been drugged for the births of all her children. She remembered very little about her labors and nothing about the births. She scarcely saw her children until they were twenty-four hours old and had to endure the pain of large episiotomies. She didn't breast-feed. She expressed regret for what she had missed and fear for her daughter, not understanding that some women could choose to have babies without drugs.

Grandma, on the other hand, was full of great stories. She had been the neighborhood midwife in her day, a casually trained assistant for her friends. She gave birth to all of her children at home, accompanied by the woman whom she worked with. She poked fun at "natural" birth, saying it was nothing new and that women had been doing it for years. She tried to reassure her daughter that Shelley knew what she was doing and just needed support and encouragement.

Grandma was a wonderful labor assistant! She rubbed Shelley's back and gave her drinks and told her how proud she was of her. Louise, in awe and still scared, sat in a chair in the corner and was afraid to participate. Shelley walked and moaned softly with each contraction. The room was quiet except for Grandma's words of encouragement. I sat with Louise, since it seemed that she needed more support than Shelley did.

I explained each step to Louise while we watched the snow fall. Shelley kept saying, "It's OK, Ma, I'm doing all right." I encouraged Louise to participate as Grandma was doing, with quiet touches and support. Soon Shelley began to make the noises of a woman ready to push, and Grandma said, "Time to call the doctor!" I checked Shelley, and she was fully dilated. I notified the doctor. Grandma smiled.

Grandma assisted Shelley to a comfortable position on the double bed, and I gathered my equipment as the doctor arrived. Shelley was pushing with her continued silent strength, and her perineum bulged before too long. The doctor applied hot soaks (gauze pads soaked in hot water) to her perineum to ease the burning of the stretch. Grandma was on one side of Shelley, and Louise had climbed onto the bed on her other side. For the first time, Louise was able to be close and touch her daughter.

The three women on the bed worked together with words and washcloths and sips of cold water. The doctor and I waited. Soon a dark hairy head emerged from Shelley's vagina, and the baby was born. A daughter. It was not yet noon. Louise was in tears, sobbing, clutching her daughter and granddaughter. Grandma sat back and smiled, observing the scene.

After the birth of the placenta and a quick check of Shelley's intact perineum and the baby, the doctor left. I left, too, to give the four generations of women some time together. As I left the room, Louise was sobbing in her mother's arms and speaking of her children's births and the regret she felt at missing such an experience. I felt honored to have shared this birth with three—now four—very special females.

Shelley and her daughter rested for a few hours and then went home with Louise and Grandma to the family's Christmas celebration. What a day it had been for everyone!

*   *   *

I tell this short, simple story for many reasons. It has always stayed in my mind as a unique experience, watching the changing moods and thoughts and actions of the women involved. This birth had been a transforming experience for all of them. It was the first birth I had attended that was peopled solely by women, and it felt so right. We all learned and shared with each other.

Older women in our culture have so much untapped wisdom. Louise had never talked with her mother about childbirth, and it had been years since Grandma had been able to participate at a birth or share what she knew. Shelley, who was trying to make a new life for herself, had come home to these women she loved and trusted, instinct letting her know that her best support was with them.

Women belong at births supporting other women. While her male partner may be important to the birthing mother, she may or may not want him there. She sometimes turns instead to her mother, sister, or close woman friend. Some women want their special women with them as well as their male partner. And many women having babies today are lesbians and have their female partner—as well as other women friends—to support them.

I have attended many births as a nurse and have also been fortunate to attend several births simply as a friend. I have found that these women wanted to spend some time in labor with me as their main support and some time with their husband or lover. The energy and the needs are very different at different stages. My own labors were the same—there were hours where I barely remember my partner's presence but instead remember the hands and words of my women friends and midwives. And then there are those times when I remember no one but him.

Labor provides us with different wants and needs at different times. We must listen to our inner voices and respond. Sometimes a woman may need to ask her male partner to leave or her woman friend, the nurse, or the midwife to stay. She may want to be alone, she may want one person there, or she may need a crowd. Her attendants need to respect her wants—and a perceptive attendant can also help a laboring woman express those needs if it seems she is holding back. Shelley was unusual because she was able to have someone in the room with her who held thoughts and feelings of fear and not of understanding. Most women would not be able to relax and open up with so much fear in the room. Grandma probably helped to guard Shelley from Louise's fear, respecting both Shelley's need to have her mother there and Louise's fear and misunderstanding.

Choice of birth companions and place to give birth are very important. A woman should think long and hard about what she wants—and she should not be afraid to change her mind if it ends up feeling not right. Hospital or home, midwife or doctor, friend, children, mother, or partner: who and where is best for you? While a birth is a special event that requires utmost care and attention, it is far from the romantic or cosmic event portrayed in so many birth stories. No woman gives birth without blood, sweat, pain, and, no doubt, a few choice curses. She needs to be in a place and with people that she can trust enough to grunt and groan and moan and swear and bleed and pee and poop and drip.

While not all women have such an easy, fast first labor and birth as Shelley did, you can be assured that her choice of companions and birth place helped to ease her work. The strength and patience of Grandma, the wonder and awe of Louise, and the respect of myself and the doctor allowed Shelley to give birth as she needed to, on a snowy Christmas morning, surrounded by the women she loved.

6

Joanne

A Planned Cesarean Birth

Joanne was pregnant with her first child. Although her pregnancy was healthy and she was excited to be having a baby, she was concerned about her past history of vaginal herpes. She had already had several lesions as she approached nine months. She knew that if she had an active lesion when she went into labor, it would be best for her to have a cesarean birth.

The day she went to the midwife for a visit in her fortieth week, she had a lesion. They cultured it to be sure; perhaps it was only a pimple. But Joanne knew—she could feel the shooting pain as the bump emerged and then the dull ache as the lesion aged. She hoped she would not go into labor until it was healed. She was also sick of being pregnant. It was a conflict, but either way she would be happy. She was looking forward to holding her child in her arms, however it was born.

Joanne and Steve had prepared for the possibility of a cesarean. They had gone to regular childbirth classes as well as a special cesarean class. They had gone to the hospital and had a tour of the operating room. They decided that Joanne would have spinal anesthesia so she could be awake for the birth, and Steve planned to be with her.

At three the next morning Joanne woke up in a puddle of fluid. Her waters had broken—the baby was not waiting for the sore to clear. She woke up Steve and called her midwife. The midwife agreed to meet her at the hospital within an hour. The midwife called the surgeon and the operating team; they would be waiting for Joanne and Steve.

Joanne was excited and did not care that she was having surgery. She was having a baby, and that fact was uppermost in her mind. The waters continued to leak as she packed and drove to the hospital. She met the midwife at the door and went to the birthing center, where she and Steve settled in to their room and prepared for surgery.

Joanne was familiar with the preparation process—signing consent forms, having an IV started, her pubic hair shaved, and a urinary catheter inserted to drain her bladder. Steve stayed with her for all the procedures, and they walked to the operating room together. Joanne had not had one contraction.

Joanne, Steve, and the midwife parted at the entrance to the operating room. Steve and the midwife went to change into scrub suits, and Joanne began her final preparations in the operating room. She was given the spinal, curled up in a ball so her back was exposed to the anesthesiologist. By the time she rolled onto her back, with numbness spreading from her feet to her chest, Steve and the midwife were at her side. The nurse washed her belly with antiseptic solution and draped her body so only her lower belly was exposed. The surgeon came into the room and spoke to her.

"All ready, Joanne? Soon your baby will be born."

Joanne smiled as the tears rolled down her cheeks. She was numb and unable to do anything other than squeeze Steve's hand. The midwife was ready with their camera as the surgery began. The surgeon spoke the entire time, explaining each step to Joanne and Steve. I waited for the birth, ready to care for the baby if there were any problems.

Soon the surgeon was down to Joanne's uterus. He made an incision and opened the organ. He reached in and lifted the baby out—a girl. Helen cried as the surgeon clamped and cut the cord and handed her to the waiting pediatrician, who brought Helen to her parents. Steve held Helen close to Joanne's face while Joanne touched her and held her hand. The midwife was busy snapping photos. The surgeon began sewing up Joanne as she and Steve admired their new daughter.

After a few minutes Joanne began to get uncomfortable and was given some medication that made her drowsy. Steve carried Helen back to their room as I trooped behind, pushing the resuscitation equipment that had been unnecessary for this birth. Helen was pink and warm, happily cuddling with her father.

Back at their room, Steve held Helen while he made phone calls—by now it was nearly dawn. I brought the scales into the room, weighed and measured Helen, and checked her vital signs. She was beautiful, well-formed, and rosy pink. I held her while Steve went for breakfast.

Soon Joanne returned. We moved her from the stretcher to the bed and cleaned her up. When she was comfortable, I handed Helen to her and helped them start nursing. After a few attempts, Helen latched on and began sucking. As I left the room, Joanne smiled at me. I could tell she was very happy.

Joanne, Steve, and Helen recovered from the surgery over the next few days. Once the spinal wore off, Joanne had her catheter removed and got out of bed. She progressed from sitting to standing to walking, and soon was getting herself to the bathroom, pushing her IV pole. Steve stayed with her and cared for Helen, changing her diapers and handing her to Joanne when she wanted to nurse. Joanne began taking liquids and then progressed to solid food. Once she was able to move well and digest her food, she was ready to leave. On Helen's fourth day of life, they all went home.

*   *   *

Cesarean birth or cesarean section? Surgery or child-birth? A nasty phrase or a welcome technology? This procedure is viewed in many ways, depending on the cir-cumstances. As the average cesarean rate moves toward 30 percent of all births in this country, it is time to look at rea-sons why this surgery is and is not necessary.

There is no need for a 30 percent cesarean rate. Since more than 90 percent of all pregnancies are uncompli-cated, that would seem to demand a cesarean rate of less than 10 percent. Some "complications" include things not related to how the baby is actually born: prematurity, for instance, or hemorrhage. The primary (first time) cesarean rate at the birthing center where I worked was 6 percent; at another hospital where I was employed, it was 25 per-cent. What was the difference?

The first important difference is that fetal monitors were not used at the birthing center. Labors were monitored by sensitive, dedicated nurses who used Doptones or feto-scopes to check on the condition of the baby. These nurses served many roles. Besides fulfilling the role of fetal moni-tor, they acted as support people, aiding the woman how-ever they could. Pain medication was rarely used: only 0.25 percent of the time (as opposed to nearly 50 percent of the labors at the other hospital). The nurses encouraged the woman in her efforts, giving her food and drink to keep up her energy, helping her walk or shower or do whatever was necessary to help her be as comfortable as possible.

Labors that slowed, stopped, or didn't start were first stimulated with nonmedical ways—herbs, castor oil, breast stimulation, orgasms, walks, discussion of fear or other psychological issues—before IV Pitocin was begun. Sometimes they worked and sometimes they didn't, but the point was that we were in no rush, had no timetable for the labor and birth, as long as mother and baby continued to be physically healthy.

In contrast, at the hospital with the 25 percent rate, women were mainly confined to bed, attached to a fetal monitor. Since the nurses felt that the monitor was doing the important work, they were rarely present, leaving the support up to a generally ill-prepared spouse. At the first sign of discomfort, they offered the woman pain medication, which was rarely refused. This group of nurses felt happier doing tasks rather than providing emotional or physical support. They also felt it was cruel to deny women pain medication and "make" them be in pain. Needless to say, these laboring women—unless they came to the hospital with a written birth plan that clearly outlined their desires for no monitor, no IV, no medication, and so on—were put on the merry-go-round right away and therefore ended up with cesareans.

Certainly there are physical reasons for having a cesarean. Placenta previa (placenta covering the cervix), placenta abruptio (placenta that comes away from the uterus before birth), footling breech (feet first), or transverse lie (sideways); severe fetal distress; and active vaginal herpes lesions are all appropriate reasons for an automatic abdominal birth. But frank breech (bottom first) position is not—although few doctors would agree with me. Many frank breech babies can be born vaginally without any problems—the key is a doctor or midwife who is well versed in vaginal breech births, who can tell if there is enough room for the baby, and who has the skills to handle any problems that may arise. Unfortunately these skills are not being taught any more, and only older general practitioners and obstetricians have enough experience. At the 25 percent hospital all breeches were born by cesarean, and most twins as well. At the birthing center most were born vaginally. Those who were born by cesarean were generally born after a trial of labor to see if a vaginal birth was possible. Of course, any woman who was uncomfortable trying a vaginal birth had the choice of a cesarean.

Most cesareans are done for "failure to progress" or "cephalopelvic disproportion"—excuses for anything from "I don't know why" to "She wasn't fast enough for me." At the birthing center the reason for these cesareans was generally mysterious—perhaps some unknown psychological holding back or an inability to let go and relax. Some were for clearly unusual fetal positions that hindered dilation. At the 25 percent hospital these cesareans were generally for women who did not follow "Friedman's curve," which dictates at what rate a woman "should" dilate. Anything off the curve is considered abnormal. Often these women had prolonged rupture of the membranes, which at the 25 percent hospital dictated that a baby must be born within twenty-four hours—or close to it—after the waters broke. The birthing center had no such policy.

Postbirth care is different depending on where one has a cesarean. At the birthing center, we encouraged the women to get up and move around as soon as possible. Although we observed carefully for signs of surgical complications, we treated women as though they had given birth instead of having had surgery. Their babies stayed in the room with them, partners were encouraged to sleep over, and the families generally went home within three or four days. At the 25 percent hospital—and others like it—the women were treated as invalids instead of new mothers and stayed a week or more. Focusing on the baby can help a woman recover sooner from her surgery and help her feel "O.K." for having had a cesarean. So often women who have had cesareans feel a sense of failure. At the birthing center there was little of that—the women *knew* they had become mothers and took on that role joyfully, aware that everything had been done to avoid their cesarean but that it had been, finally, necessary.

Joanne and Steve were happy to have had a cesarean birth. They did not want to take the chance of infecting their newborn with the herpes virus. They chose a cesarean for the birth of their second child because the virus was once again present. The important word for Joanne and Steve was "choice." No one forced them to do something they did not want to do. But for too many women across this country having a cesarean is hardly a choice. It is too often a painful end to a natural process that was interfered with by paranoid and inflexible birth attendants. The way to avoid that scenario is to educate yourself, have a detailed birth plan, and choose a birth place and attendants who will genuinely support you and respect your wishes. You should demand nothing less.

7

Laura

Infection, Induction, and Intensive Care

Laura was thirty-five weeks pregnant with her first baby when her waters broke. After twenty-four hours she had not gone into labor and was admitted to the hospital. We had a conservative prolonged rupture of the membranes (PROM) policy: no inducing labor, just a "wait and watch" attitude.

Laura and her husband, Mark, settled themselves into a birthing room. Laura's temperature and pulse, as well as the baby's heartbeat, were checked every four hours, and her blood was drawn once a day. We were checking for signs of infection, at which time induction would be necessary. In this situation, most women went into labor on their own within three or four days and gave birth to healthy babies.

Mark went to work every day while Laura watched TV, read, and walked the halls. The nurses enjoyed having her around to talk with when things were quiet. Laura liked being with everyone, feeling the casual and comfortable atmosphere of the place. It helped her to relax and prepare for whatever was ahead—having her baby early was not something she had planned on!

Four days after her waters broke, Laura began to show

signs of infection—a rising white blood cell count and slight fever. The induction would begin. Laura and Mark were excited that their baby would be born soon.

Laura was not dilated at all when the intravenous (IV) was started. She had been examined by the cleanest method possible, sterile speculum. The fluid still coming out of her was clear, and a sample was sent to the lab to be checked for organisms. Pitocin was added to the piggy-back IV, and the drug began to run into her veins. It was four in the afternoon.

Starting a Pitocin induction from scratch is a long process. It takes a while for the uterus to begin its work. I increased the dosage every fifteen minutes and checked the baby's heartbeat as often. Laura and Mark and their doctor were playing cards. It was a relaxed time; Laura barely noticed the small twinges emanating from her uterus. I worked until eleven that night, when the night shift nurse took over. We had spent the evening with the TV on, playing many games of cards, and waiting. I knew it would be a long night for Laura and Mark.

When I returned the next morning at seven, I found Laura and Mark a little blurry from lack of sleep. Laura's contractions had remained five minutes apart and mild through most of the night. They were able to catch a few winks in between. By six o'clock the contractions had become stronger, and Laura was finally in active labor.

That morning Laura alternated walking with rests in bed and showers. She remained strong, and subsequent blood tests and vital sign readings did not show any further infection. Laura and her baby were doing the best job they could, and it was a great one. Moving around helped Laura work with the contractions, and at 11 A.M. she said she had to push.

Laura's first vaginal exam confirmed her feeling, and she began pushing. She gave birth half an hour later to her daughter, Catherine. Catherine was slow to breathe, but with some stimulation and cuddling on her mother's belly, she recovered well and was pink and lusty at five minutes of age. But five minutes later she turned dusky, and I gave her some oxygen. Then she began to breathe with marked difficulty, and I took her to the special nursery.

Laura birthed her placenta and received a few stitches for a small perineal tear. When she was clean and settled, Mark came out to the nursery to check on Catherine. Catherine was in an isolette, receiving oxygen. The clear plastic box was heated to keep her warm and enclosed to keep the proper oxygen concentration. I had my hands through the portholes and was holding her, trying to reassure her in this early stressful time. I showed Mark how to put his hands through the portholes, and he stroked and calmed her.

The pediatrician soon arrived, and the laborious task of testing Catherine for her problem began. We drew blood for cell counts and oxygen content. She was not pinking up or breathing any easier in her warm, oxygen-rich environment. She had chest X rays and a spinal tap. Mark went back and forth between Laura and Catherine, caring for them both.

Soon we had a diagnosis of pneumonia, and Catherine was started on antibiotics. She still struggled with her breathing but seemed to relax in the warmth of the isolette. She slept a great deal but periodically opened her eyes to look at her surroundings. She had a nurse by her side constantly, for reassurance and safety. She had many wires attached to her: heartbeat and breathing monitors, temperature check, and IV tubing. Laura wanted to see her but was afraid of all the equipment.

That evening Mark finally convinced Laura to see Catherine. He brought her down in a wheelchair; Laura was feeling too weak to walk, and she was afraid of fainting when she saw Catherine. Laura began to cry when she saw her daughter, who was laboring with each breath and was attached to so many wires. Mark showed Laura how to put her hands through the portholes and touch Catherine. It was a scene that would repeat itself many times over the years: a mother's first look, again, at her child who had been gone from her side for some time.

Catherine continued to be quite sick and needed constant supervision for three days. Laura pumped her breasts and saved her milk for the time when Catherine would be ready to suckle. Laura's strength came back, and she gradually began to spend more and more time with Catherine, changing her diapers, making her comfortable, holding her hand. After four days, Catherine came out of the isolette, and her parents were able to hold her. In a week she was nursing well, and was free of her illness, and the family went home.

I continued to be friends with Laura and Mark. Laura vowed she would never have another child; she felt the whole experience had been too traumatic for her and Catherine. She did not want that to happen again. But in time, as with so many women, the memory of labor and birth became fuzzy and distant, and Laura was pregnant again. Much to her surprise, she gave birth over an intact perineum to a full-term, healthy baby boy after three hours of labor. Whoever expected that all labors should be the same?

*   *   *

What happened the first time? Why did Laura's waters break five weeks early, and why did Catherine develop pneumonia? No one knows. This is one of the great continuing mysteries of childbirth. Where does the signal come from that it is time to be born? Why at one time and not another? Perhaps this will continue to be a mystery even in this age of advancing reproductive technology. So many doctors are involved in manipulating the process from beginning to end and deciding through the use of technology when the "best time" is for birth. Hopefully this one true mystery can remain so.

And who's to say that babies know best? Why did Laura's waters break five weeks early? Why did Catherine want to be born then? And if she had wanted to be born then, why didn't Laura go into labor on her own? We had not encouraged Laura and Mark to try alternative methods of induction because it was still, theoretically, too early for Catherine to be born: the possibility of complications of prematurity were there—low birth weight, respiratory difficulties, jaundice.

Childbirth is eminently spiritual and practical. We could spend years discussing the whys of so many things: why some babies are born very early, some late, some headfirst, some bottom first, some without a care in the world, some with life-threatening deformities. Some of these things can be attributed to physical factors, but more often than not, there is no answer.

For some women, this answerless state is deeply troubling; others take it as part of what life dishes out. Some women feel they have "failed" if their baby is not born the way they had "planned"; other women plan nothing at all. Even birth attendants are amazed and awed by the events surrounding childbirth, often too busy to wonder why. But then the questions come back to haunt us: why one woman can have a fifteen-minute labor while another struggles for days and days, why one baby suffering from meconium aspiration dies and another lives.

Perhaps that is part of the uniqueness that draws people to childbirth, the mixture of the predictable and unpredictable. People who need to control things in their lives— whether they are doctors, nurses, midwives, or pregnant women—seem to have a harder time with this mysterious aspect of childbearing.

Laura and Mark were practical people, deeply in love, with no expectations other than wanting to have a child in their lives. Catherine's prematurity and illness took them both by surprise, but they involved themselves in what was happening in their own time, in their own way. Laura was very comfortable in the hospital, yet Mark was more comfortable being with Catherine in the more unknown atmosphere of the special nursery. A mother's vulnerability or a father's practicality? As with so many things, there is no answer.

For birth attendants the lesson is clear. Discussions with parents like Laura and Mark are paramount—answering their questions, explaining the various tests, personnel, and equipment that will be entering their lives. Continuing to be patient with explanations, demonstrations, and encouragement to help them through this strange and unexpected time. Staying with the baby and filling in until the parents are able to take over, providing the baby with the physical closeness she needs and craves.

Complications such as this one need not change a birth into a high-tech experience. A conservative PROM policy usually allows a woman to give birth at her own pace; inductions because of possible infections are rarely necessary. When they are, the woman can still birth her baby without excessive intervention: no need for a fetal monitor if a nurse stays with her, no need for a delivery table or an episiotomy, and infant resuscitation equipment can be available at the bedside, if needed, as well as oxygen and a heated bed.

Certainly parents want their baby born in what they feel is the safest environment. Families also want to maintain their sense of togetherness and the feeling that birth is a family event. By discussing the pros and cons of various technologies and interventions as well as answering questions along the way, safety *and* togetherness can each have its place. Then the birth of the child will be the beginning of a family—not the beginning of a complicated medical event. *Women* give birth: it's up to the attendants to respect each woman's place as the mother of the baby and not as a bystander watching nurse as mother and doctor as savior.

Sick baby or healthy baby, each one deserves our respect and love. The baby has made a journey and has to use all its strength to fight the germs that have invaded its body. The baby needs all the love, encouragement, and physical contact it can get to recover, as well as antibiotics, oxygen, and a warm environment. Likewise, the mother needs love as well as encouragement to help her discover that she has the strength to give birth and care for her child even under adversity.

8

Karen

A Five-Day Labor

It was midnight and the night was quiet. At the birthing center, there were two women and babies who were planning to leave in the morning. I settled in with a good book to pass the hours until one of the women needed me. It was snowy and cold, nearing the holidays.

A phone call broke the peacefulness; the admitting desk was calling to tell me a woman had arrived in labor. Karen and Bob, a couple in their mid-thirties, walked in as I hung up the phone. They were cheerful despite an hour's drive through the snow. They were excited to be having their first baby.

They sat with me and we chatted. Karen did not want to get undressed or go to a room, she wanted to talk and she wanted to hear the baby's heartbeat. I got out the Dop-tone, she lifted her shirt, and I placed the device on her abdomen. The clear thump-thump-thump echoed throughout the room. The baby sounded fine.

By 2 A.M. Karen was fading and wanted to rest. Her contractions were short and irregular: some five minutes apart, others three, seven, or even ten. She only had to close her eyes and relax during them and seemed very peaceful, but I knew they weren't very strong—it was early yet. I settled Karen and Bob into one of the rooms, where they stretched out on the bed together and cuddled.

A few hours later Bob came out to get me. He said that the contractions were stronger and that Karen was having a hard time dealing with them. I went to their room and sat with them. Karen was sitting cross-legged on the bed, still with a cheerful look, but seemed to struggle more when a contraction came. The contractions were more regular now—about five minutes apart—but still mild to my palpation.

Karen asked me to do a vaginal exam; she was two centimeters dilated, and her cervix was still thick. She had a long way to go. I knew her doctor would send her home come daylight, with instructions to have a long hot bath and a couple of glasses of wine and get some sleep. Hard instructions to hear when you are as excited as Karen was to be having a baby—but sometimes necessary.

Karen was in prodromal labor, very early labor that can last for several days. These contractions usually just soften up the cervix in preparation for the stronger contractions that will open it all the way. Some birth attendants call it "piddling around," but whatever the name, it is not an easy time—for the woman, her partner, or their birth attendant. The woman often gets frustrated and upset at the length of time without clear progress. Her partner isn't sure how to help, and the attendant is often bombarded with phone call after phone call asking for help.

When their doctor arrived at 7 A.M., he checked Karen; she was still two centimeters dilated, and he sent them home with the bath and wine advice. They were not to return until the contractions were three minutes apart and one minute long. I could see the sadness behind their cheerful faces as they left for the long drive home.

The next night the same scene repeated itself. This time Karen was three centimeters dilated, but she hadn't slept or eaten for thirty-six hours. She was exhausted.

After she was given a small dose of morphine, Karen slept peacefully for three hours. She had some toast and yogurt and said she felt a little better. The contractions continued, three minutes apart and one minute long but very mild. At 6 A.M. the doctor came to see Karen and Bob. He taught Bob how to do a vaginal exam to check for dilation. After giving them a good supply of sterile gloves and a cervical dilation chart, he sent Bob and Karen home again, with instructions to return when Karen was five centimeters dilated.

Other laboring women came in, had their babies, and left. We wondered what had happened to Karen and Bob. Two days later they returned, triumphant. Karen was now five centimeters dilated, and they knew they had reached the final stretch.

Karen walked and showered and rested, exhausted because she had not slept since the morphine dose two days before. We encouraged her to drink plenty of fluids, but she was not interested in eating. Her contractions still were not that strong, but they were regular, and she continued to dilate. Karen had remarkable stamina and good cheer. Where any other woman probably would have folded days before, she was still optimistic.

About midnight Karen was six centimeters dilated—four days after she and Bob had first arrived at the birthing center. After some discussion, Karen decided that she would like to have her waters broken with the possibility that the procedure might speed up her labor.

At 7 A.M. Karen was seven centimeters dilated, at noon she was eight centimeters, by four in the afternoon she was completely dilated and ready to push. Throughout all of this the baby was fine: steady heartbeat, no sign of infection or other stress.

Karen tried various positions for pushing, but after two hours had made little progress. The baby seemed to be in a good position but was probably in the nine-pound range. Karen and Bob decided, after discussion with the doctor and nurse, that starting an IV with some Pitocin would be a good idea. Karen's uterus was getting tired: the fluid would give Karen extra energy at a time she needed it most, and the Pitocin would help increase the strength of the contractions. The possibility of hemorrhage was increased because of the amount of time Karen had been in labor; a tired uterus often does not respond well after a birth, and there was the danger that she might bleed too much.

The IV and the Pitocin were started, and Karen resumed pushing. The drug seemed to work, or perhaps the energy in the fluid was helping, and Karen began to make some progress. By 6 P.M. the baby's head was visible during pushes, and a half hour later the baby was born—a healthy ten-pound boy. Karen birthed her placenta easily, received a couple of stitches for a small tear, and settled in to nurse Joshua. It had been five days since she had had her first contraction.

Karen, Bob, and Joshua stayed a couple of days to rest and get used to each other. Karen, as cheerful as ever, walked the hall with Joshua in the wee hours of the morning. She seemed unfazed by her ordeal. She ate hearty meals and slept as much as possible. We asked her if she felt it was worth it, knowing that in another place she would have had the Pitocin started sooner and an increased chance for a cesarean. Karen said she was very pleased with her treatment and that her main concern was that she had been frustrated about being sent home. But now, with her son in her arms, she regretted nothing.

*   *   *

But *was* it worth it? Would Karen suffer at home? Would the exhaustion catch up with her? Would she have a long recovery and the possibility of postpartum complications such as infection or depression? Would other birthing professionals say we were just lucky that Joshua was fine and that Karen didn't hemorrhage or develop an infection during labor? The staff mulled this labor over, the longest we had experienced, wondering if we had done the right thing, wondering if we had helped or hurt Karen and her family. Had it been easy to sit back and let nature take her course because Karen had been so cheerful? Had we been right to send them home twice and to teach Bob to do vaginal exams?

Most hospitals would not have allowed this to happen. Karen would have had her waters broken and/or Pitocin started that first morning, and the baby would have been born within twenty-four hours (more likely sixteen). Her chance for a cesarean, or at least forceps, would have been great. And would that have been so wrong or so bad for everyone involved?

My major complaint with that scenario is that the decision-making power would probably be left up to the professionals, without discussion with and *permission* from Karen and Bob. Most likely they would have been told what was happening, with the IV started while the nurse or doctor was explaining Pitocin to them. Or her waters would have been broken during a vaginal exam with no more discussion than the warning "This won't hurt, things will just be warm and wet."

At our birthing center, Karen and Bob were involved in the decision-making process the whole time. And although Karen said she didn't like being sent home, she understood that her chances for relaxation, sleep, and progress were probably greater at home than in the hospital. Plus, Karen and Bob had no health insurance and were trying their best to keep costs down. (At our birthing center only a nominal fee was charged for women in early labor who stayed less than eight hours.) No move was made without a complete discussion of all the pros and cons, and Karen and Bob's approval. In fact, Pitocin had been discussed several times before Karen and Bob decided it was a good idea.

For many women, the experience of "piddling around"

is frustrating. They know they are in labor, yet nothing seems to be happening. They get tired and angry or scared or unsure of themselves. They feel embarrassed by frequent calls or visits to their birth attendant. They wonder if it's time to go to the hospital or time to call the midwife to their home. They lose trust in their bodies and their strength to give birth. While this early labor activity is certainly common, especially with first babies, it by no means guarantees five days of labor with virtually no sleep or food—two or three days is more usual.

This is a good example of the necessity to eat and rest as much as possible during early labor. While long walks, lovemaking, and various herbal remedies may be useful to encourage labor to be more active, it is also important for a woman to keep up her strength and spirit. Aggressive stimulating techniques may only make her more tired and tense. In some cases it may be better to let nature take her course. By being in the place most comfortable to her, usually at home, and with those people surrounding her whom she trusts, a woman may be more apt to relax and allow things to happen.

There are many women like Karen—slow and steady wins the race—but at what cost? Will women feel guilty and tense up if they are afraid they aren't performing on schedule when their labors take longer than the textbook twelve or fourteen hours? (And since when do women worry or feel bad about themselves if they have a *shorter-than-average* labor?) Will they feel their body is failing them? Will they worry for the safety of their baby? Will they simply give up and not care any more? Or will they do as one woman did—rip out the IV and demand a cesarean ASAP (as soon as possible), even though she was progressing and seemed to be relaxed and coping with her labor?

As an added aside and more food for thought, when Karen had her second child three years later, she opted for starting the Pitocin sooner when the same pattern began to develop, and after twelve hours of "slow" progress, she asked for, and received, a cesarean. She gave birth to a twelve-pound girl and went home in two days, well rested and cheerful. Which experience was better for her and her children? Does it matter? Is the main point that Karen *chose* her two birth experiences and accepted full responsibility for them? I believe it is.

Karen and Bob's story illustrates another aspect of the differences that occur during the birthing process. Textbooks and childbirth classes are full of "facts" about labor lengths, progression or dilation in terms of hours per centimeter, so many hours or minutes of pushing, average birth weight, the "normalcy" of episiotomy, post-placenta Pitocin, no food during labor, fetal monitors, and so on ad infinitum. What books and classes *should* be discussing is the wonderful rainbow of differences from one woman to the next. Childbirth is no place for schedules and routines; it is one experience that is completely out of the realm of averages and should be treated as such.

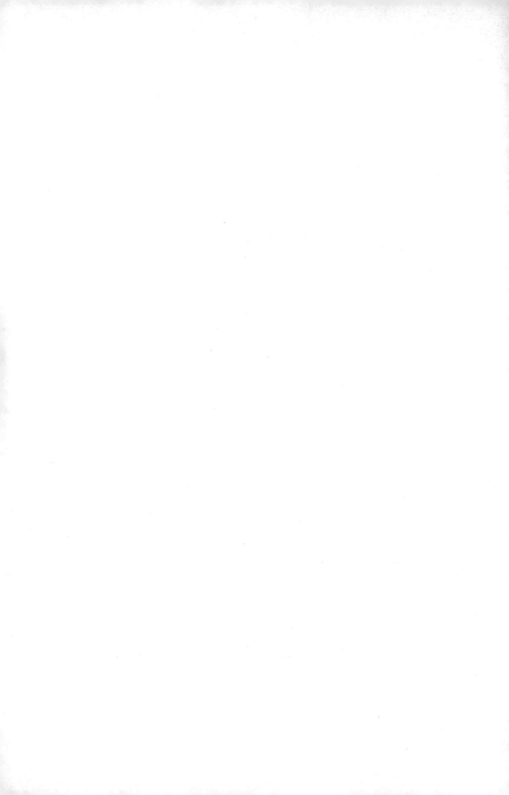

9

Hannah

Joyful Home Birth

It was a cold fall morning when I was called by Mike, father of two, soon to be father of three. His partner, Hannah, had been having mild contractions for a few hours, and her waters had just broken. They were an hour away. It was time to go.

I drove rapidly through the foggy morning and thought about Hannah and Mike and their two kids, Tom and Sarah, who had both been born at home, in the same cabin, far up in the hills. This baby was luckier: it was September, rather than January, when Tom and Sarah had been born. No fear of snow or ice on this day.

When I arrived at their home, Mike was cooking a big breakfast of pancakes for everyone. Hannah was walking around. Tom, six, was drawing pictures. Sarah, four, was looking at books. Soon all of us—Hannah included—sat down to steaming stacks of pancakes with applesauce and maple syrup.

After breakfast Mike and Hannah went for a walk, the kids continued to play, and I relaxed with a book. Soon the doctor arrived, and I filled her in on what was happening. Tom and Sarah crowded around, showing us their pictures and books. It seemed a regular morning for them, with the addition of a couple more adults available to play with.

It was midmorning when Hannah and Mike returned from their walk. The contractions were still irregular and mild, and Hannah was still leaking clear fluid. They decided to turn to their tried-and-true labor-inducing technique: breast stimulation. Hannah's last labor had had a similar slow start, and not too long after enjoying some breast stimulation, she had gone into active labor and given birth to Sarah.

The doctor and I continued to play baby-sitter; Tom and Sarah were curious and asked questions about what was happening with their mom, but they also seemed to be very calm about the impending arrival. We continued to talk together, read books, and play.

Fifteen or twenty minutes had passed when we heard soft but insistent breathing coming from upstairs. We ventured to the bottom of the stairs and asked how things were going. Before Hannah could answer, she had another contraction, clutching the railing, squatting, and breathing with a low and regular moan. She emerged from the contraction smiling and said, "It's really happening now!"

Tom and Sarah shyly followed us to the stairs, and soon the four of us made our way to the bedroom to join Hannah and Mike. The doctor listened to the baby's heartbeat while I set up the birthing equipment. Tom and Sarah got reassuring hugs from their parents, and they climbed onto the bed to wait, talking quietly together and looking out the window at the beautiful fall morning.

A few contractions later, Hannah's breathing changed with the distinctive sound of a woman ready to push, and she moved to the bed. Propped up with pillows and supported by Mike, Hannah began to push. Tom and Sarah gradually moved closer to their mother as we all encouraged her in her efforts. Between pushes Mike and Hannah talked with Tom and Sarah about their roles in the impending birth; Tom decided to hold the flashlight and Sarah, the mirror. The feeling in the room was very relaxed, and Hannah was smiling more often than not. After one long push Hannah leaned back and said, "I just love having babies."

Tom and Sarah's eyes grew bigger as they watched the baby begin to emerge, and in no time they were beside their parents, looking at their sister, Tillie. The new family was wrapped in warm, dry blankets, the cord was cut, and the placenta was born. The doctor and I cleaned up and went downstairs to leave parents and children alone together, sounds of giggles and exclamations coming from the bedroom.

"If only every birth could be so easy," we commented as we relaxed in the living room. After a little while, we returned to the new family to check on Hannah's bleeding and to do Tillie's physical exam. A couple of hours later, after everyone was checked and settled, we left to return to our busy lives. It was barely afternoon on that glorious, crisp autumn day.

* * *

Why is it that some women have such a (seemingly) easy time and others struggle for days on end, exhausted from lack of sleep? Perhaps it is just another of life's mysteries—are labor length and intensity physically based, are they psychological, or, more likely, some combination of the two? Everyone's pain perception is different, some people are generally more relaxed and accepting, and clearly every labor is different. Even one woman's labors are not necessarily the same: short one time, long the next, slow and exhausting, or quick and painfully intense.

While Hannah seems to be one of the "lucky" ones, there are probably several factors contributing to her ease of giving birth. She was giving birth in the place she loved the most, the place where she had *chosen* to give birth.

Having chosen three home births, it was clear that this was a well-thought-out decision for Hannah and Mike. Having their children participate was equally a planned choice. Having accepting and respectful birth attendants contributed to Hannah's relaxation. Hannah was a woman who accepted her body, its strengths and weaknesses, its size, and its power. And yet, even for other women who have these important factors present, their labors are not as brief or as seemingly painless as Hannah's. And so we return to the physical as well as the psychological.

Every woman, except those with a few specific physical conditions, is capable of giving birth vaginally. But for every woman that means something different. Some women may have slowly building contractions over several days and then push for hours, others may have strong contractions from the onset for several hours and then give birth in one push, still others may have an hour or two of contractions until they are fully dilated and then may push equally long. Perhaps part of the mystery of birth is that one never knows what will happen and that each labor has to be taken individually, with no expectations.

Tillie's birth was also special because of the participation of her brother and sister. One does not have to have a home birth to have sibling participation. Many hospitals will allow children at the birth, usually if they are accompanied by an adult who can attend to their needs and explain things to them. I have seen hundreds of siblings from age two to sixteen witness the birth of their baby brother or sister, and without exception, they have been positive experiences. Depending on their age and level of preparation, they participated at different levels—from sitting in a chair in the corner, watching silently, to holding their mother and encouraging her while she was in the shower attempting to relax.

I have often surmised that father participation at birth

may reduce future child abuse. I also suspect that sibling participation at birth reduces the amount of culturally expected jealousy of the new baby. When a child can experience the wonder of birth (and that is usually what makes the strongest impression—the blood and noise mean little to them) and get a chance to bond with the new sibling right away, I think that he or she feels more a part of the baby's life. The baby is not something inflicted upon them when it returns home from the hospital but is clearly a part of a whole from the start. The theory of mother-infant bonding is expanded to include all members of the family.

Of course, there are many choices, and children should not be forced to attend a birth it they do not want to or if the laboring woman is not comfortable with the idea. But perhaps they can be close by and can come into the room soon after the baby is born. Often a birth happens in the middle of the night, when a child is sleeping, or a woman is uncomfortable baring her body in front of her child. In any case, actually participating in a long labor may be too much for any child, but with a supportive adult in attendance, a sibling can while away the hours playing, reading, eating, or sleeping and come into the room at the time of birth.

Place of birth and sibling participation are just two of the many choices that parents must make when a baby is expected. As with all the other factors, such as type of birth attendant, use of technology, laboring positions, and postpartum care, the important issue is that women and their partners make a *choice* as to what is best for them—not just have things happen to them at the comfort level of those in attendance. A birth belongs to the parents, who should welcome their new family member in a way that is best for them.

10

Mary

Childbirth and Violence
Against Women

Mary was an "elderly primip" (thirty-eight years old and expecting her first child). I was a nursing student. I was assigned to watch Mary's labor and, if I was lucky, her birth. I had gone to nursing school with plans to become a midwife. Finally, at long last, I was to help someone in labor. I was nervous and excited and very, very happy.

I was led into the small, windowless labor room by my nursing instructor and introduced to Mary and her husband, John. They hardly had time to give their permission for me to stay; the contractions were coming fast and furious. Mary looked very uncomfortable in the narrow bed; the walls were covered with equipment of various kinds, and John was sandwiched between the head of the bed and the fetal monitor. A nurse was busy trying to get the monitor to work as Mary thrashed around, forced to lie on her back in a tiny, crowded room full of strangers.

Besides myself, the nurse, Mary, and John, there was a coterie of interns and medical students eager to be part of the action. Some were intent on the monitor; others were intent on what the chief resident was telling them about

Mary's case. I made myself as small as possible at the foot of the bed, maintaining direct eye contact with Mary.

Mary and John had tried to conceive for many years and had finally given up. They were well established in their careers when this surprise pregnancy came along. Mary had had all the appropriate prenatal care, genetic testing, and childbirth classes. John and Mary wanted natural childbirth for their first, and probably only, child. Mary had hooked herself up with the specialists at the big medical center and felt comfortable that they would provide her with a healthy, happy baby.

But, in the present, Mary's contractions were coming every two to three minutes and lasting sixty to ninety seconds. There was little rest in between. Her labor had begun at seven that morning, and now it was 10 A.M. The residents were preparing the students and the couple for a long, hard day; after all, this was her first baby and she was so "old." Without asking or preparing her, the doctor did a vaginal exam. Mary practically leapt off the bed.

After announcing to the audience that Mary was eight centimeters dilated, the doctor asked for an amnihook and broke Mary's bag of waters. No word of explanation, certainly not asking her permission; he just did it. The warm, clear fluid rushed out of Mary, went all over the bed, and dripped onto the floor. The nurse looked dismayed and Mary looked even more scared, a prisoner in the bed. The doctor patted her patronizingly, told her she was progressing nicely, and left the room.

As the nurse hustled to change the sheets before the next event could happen, the anesthesiologist walked in and asked Mary if she'd like "a little something" to take away the pain. Mary looked questioningly at her husband and then said no, she was doing all right, and things seemed to be going fast anyway.

The anesthesiologist kept pressing her, but Mary held her ground. He hung around for a few minutes, checking the printout from the monitor and generally hassling the nurse, who already seemed pretty hassled. She had so many tasks set before her by the insensitive medical staff that she had no time to speak with Mary or John. After complaining to the nurse one last time about the quality of the monitor printout and unsuccessfully pressuring Mary again, the anesthesiologist left the room.

The next half hour was calmer as medical students wandered in and out, exposing Mary's crotch with each swoosh of the curtain, and the nurse got things tidied up. The attendants attended the monitor, watching it, adjusting it, commenting on it. Mary and John did the best they could—she breathed, in a fashion, with the contractions; he had a cool washcloth and ice chips at the ready. Mary's requests for something to drink, a change of position, and a cover over her legs were all refused.

Mary and I kept up eye contact, and John was still stuck behind her, able to communicate only by a hand on her forehead or shoulder. She was getting more and more uncomfortable and was valiantly trying to keep up, despite her circumstances. A few contractions later, I saw a new look in her eyes and heard a change in her breathing—she had to push.

Doctors and nurses and more doctors checked her, just to make sure she was fully dilated. How could that be so? It was much too soon! The nurse, and another, rushed off to set up the delivery room. Another nurse came in to remove John so that he could change his clothes. The doctors were in and out, off to scrub. They patted Mary and said, "It won't be long now, dear, just relax."

Just relax! Mary was panic-stricken. Where once there had been a room teeming with people, she was now left alone with me.

"Is everything OK? Am I OK? Is the baby OK? What's going on?" she asked in a weak, scared voice. I answered the best I could before I, too, was whisked away by a nurse who instructed me to scrub and don gown, booties, cap, and mask. I turned around, and Mary flew by me on a gurney, screaming. I entered the delivery room and stood in the corner near the foot of the table.

Mary screamed with each contraction and attempted to push. There was no one to coach her; the nurses were still setting up and the doctors were scrubbing. The fetal monitor had been abandoned in the labor room. Mary yelled for water, for help, for her husband. The anesthesiologist came into the room and asked her if she was now ready for something to take away the pain. "Yes, oh, yes," she cried.

The next fifteen minutes were filled with the anesthesiologist attempting to give Mary an epidural. But Mary was so scared and lost and confused that she squirmed constantly, and finally two nurses had to hold her in place before the needle found its mark. Mary sighed with relief and lay back on the table.

Now John was seated at her head and the doctor told her to start pushing. Mary stared at him in confusion. Push? How was she to do that? There was no sensation, no guidance at all. The doctor began to yell at her and told her to hurry up and do her part. Push! Push! Mary made some gallant efforts, and the doctor, in his frustration, spoke to the nurse.

"Get me the suction setup," he ordered.

The nurse procured the necessary sterile supplies, after hurriedly pushing me out of the way. The doctor busied himself with hooking things up and telling Mary that he would help her, since she didn't seem to be able to do it herself.

The vacuum extractor whirred to life, and the doctor placed the cap on the baby's head. Mary winced with the pressure, and the doctor told her to lie still. After a few moments the doctor told her to push. He pulled, and the cap popped off. The doctor had been pulling so hard that he nearly fell to the floor. This charade went on for the next fifteen minutes while I watched in horror. I never saw anyone check the baby's heartbeat in all that time—the nurses were too busy trying to help the doctor get the machine to work properly.

Finally the suction cup seemed to stick, and the baby descended with the assistance of the doctor's manly strength. He cut a huge episiotomy that extended through Mary's rectum with the birth of her son. The baby was dangled in the air, the cord was cut, and he was handed to the pediatrician, who removed him to the heated bed in the corner. Mary and John were ecstatic, I was crying, and the doctor was telling Mary to hold still so he could stitch her up. The repair took so long that John and the baby finally left with the pediatric staff to go to the nursery. I was left with the fuming doctor, the circulating nurse, and Mary, who was in a drug-induced sleep. She had been given an intravenous painkiller during the repair, and so they worked in silence, oblivious to the woman who had just become a mother.

I stayed with Mary in the recovery room and helped her on the postpartum ward the next couple of days. She was in a great deal of pain from her episiotomy and she was worried about her "conehead" son with the big, purple bruise on his head. I did my best to reassure her that time would heal all, and that she and her baby would be normal again. I had a hard time answering her questions and listening to her concerns about the labor and birth. She realized that horrible things had happened and that something had been taken away from her. She also felt grateful to the doctor, who had "done his best." I could only listen without responding.

* * *

Mary's experience is not unusual. She got on the merry-go-round and was powerless to get off. She did not have the tools or the strength at such a vulnerable time. John was in no position to help, either. Mary had no support from the nurses, who were too busy responding to the doctors' orders or messing around with the machinery (monitor, vacuum extractor, delivery room setup). The doctors had their own agendas, which included making money, doing things their own way, and getting through as fast as possible. But mostly this story illustrates a very insidious form of violence against women.

Everyone is familiar with domestic violence and the commonness with which women are abused in their own homes by a trusted husband or lover. But violence against women occurs at all levels of society and in many unexpected places. Doctors, lawyers, and corporate executives are known to abuse their wives as well as their patients or clients. In fact, according to statistics, it is just those men who are the majority of batterers, along with police and military officers.

A common educational tool used in working with battered women is the "Power and Control Wheel." This diagram, a wheel with eight spokes, shows the numerous ways that batterers maintain power and control over their victims. In addition to physical violence, the spokes that hold the wheel together are emotional abuse, economic abuse, sexual abuse, using children, threats, using male privilege, intimidation, and isolation. Mary's story illustrates all of these points.

Emotional abuse involves actions that make a woman feel bad about herself or make her feel crazy. By performing procedures without asking or explaining them, by telling a woman to "get in control" or that she is gaining too much weight, the doctor is abusing her.

Economic abuse is harder to pin down in this particular situation, but we all know that doctors and hospitals charge way too much for their services and often order tests and procedures just to make money from them. And, clearly, women who do not have health insurance are constantly being abused.

Sexual abuse is rampant in doctors' offices across the country. Anytime a vaginal exam is done without a woman's permission, she is being sexually abused. Any passing comments about the attractiveness or unattractiveness of a woman's genitalia or breasts can also be considered abusive. A woman's body is her own, and no physician (or other person) has the right to touch her without her permission.

Using children is a classic way to abuse women. An abusive husband will often threaten to take the kids away or report her to child protective services—anything to make her feel guilty so he can keep control over her. A doctor will tell a woman she is hurting her unborn child if she refuses any tests or procedures that he thinks are necessary.

Threats are commonplace—threatening Pitocin induction or cesarean section, threatening to give her pain medication against her will if she does not get "in control" and "cooperate." Threatening, threatening, threatening—tests, procedures, damaged infants—all as a way to control her, to allow him to do what *he* wants, what makes *him* feel comfortable.

Using *male privilege* is a cornerstone of our society. Men are not alone here; many women doctors do the same things, relying on "physician privilege": the right to order nurses, lab techs, secretaries, and patients around. This shows up as a general attitude of "I'm right and you're wrong. I know more than you. I am the doctor. I am God." A doctor who does not allow a woman any part in decision making is exerting his male privilege and is abusing her right as a person to make her own choices.

Intimidation is also common, based on much of the same privilege and godlike status: "I know more than you do, so you better do as I say." Using looks or comments to put

women in a place of fear: "I'll give you another half-hour
to get to ten centimeters, or I'm afraid I'll have to section
you, dear. You're not progressing on schedule."

And finally there is *isolation*, a common problem in almost any hospital situation. Family and friends are often
kept from the laboring woman. Visiting hours are at certain times, some hospital emergency rooms don't allow
parents to accompany sick or injured children into the
exam rooms, and on maternity and labor and delivery
floors, husbands and partners are considered dirty and in
the way. If they are to be tolerated at all, they must behave;
sit or stand in the right place; and wear the proper clothing. Extended family, dear friends, and children are rarely
allowed to be with the woman as she gives birth. Isolation
is both physical and mental; lack of information about
what is happening also constitutes abuse.

Could things have been different for Mary? Of course
they could. There are those few-and far-between physicians, midwives, and hospitals that step back and watch a
woman give birth as she chooses, with support as necessary. Mary and her husband could have labored and given
birth in a comfortable room, with plenty of space to walk
and move, a window to the outside world, chairs and a
comfortable bed, a bathroom in the room, and some privacy from medical and nursing students. Mary could have
labored in the position of her choice, without the hassles
of being attached to the fetal monitor. A sensitive nurse or
midwife could have listened to the baby's heartbeat at regular intervals with a Doptone or fetoscope, and could have
offered food, drink, and encouragement as necessary.

When Mary felt the urge to push, one of her attendants
could have done a vaginal exam, with her permission, and
then could have discussed the pros and cons of breaking
her waters, getting Mary's permission before doing anything. Mary could have been assisted to push in a squatting position or on the toilet or in another position that she
found comfortable and useful. At the time of the birth,

Mary could have found a good position somewhere in the room without having to be moved; she could have been guided to birth the head gently without tearing, and could have reached down and lifted her son up onto her belly, where he could have been held by his mother while suctioned, dried, and observed as necessary. John would never have left her side, and the two parents could have completely enjoyed the experience of seeing and holding their son as soon as he was born. And, most important, Mary could have survived the experience intact, with a greater sense of self-esteem and empowerment than she had before she went into labor.

Why is this so hard for some doctors and nurses to do? Because *they would lose control.* The power balance needs to shift from the medical staff to the woman and her family, where it rightly belongs. The medical staff should simply observe and assist, leaving the decision making and the choices to the family. But doctors and nurses cannot stand to lose control of their power, their procedures, their routines. When asked "why" about questionable and outdated procedures, many medical personnel are known to say "Because we've always done it that way," without consideration that times may have changed and that there may be a better, simpler, more sensible way.

In many ways, this is a classic birth horror story. Not all births are like this. But in many places a pregnant family has to be wary and prepare themselves for such possibilities. Doing your research while pregnant is very important; check out your choice of doctor, midwife, and hospital before you go into labor. A written birth plan may be absolutely necessary as a way to protect yourself. For those who have the option, shopping around may provide the best answer. Many hospitals are now realizing that it is good business to provide consumers with what they want. Do not stop searching and planning until your choice feels 100 percent comfortable to you.

Education, support, and planning are the keys to help a

battered woman get out, and stay out, of an abusive relationship. A pregnant woman and her family can learn all
that there is about pregnancy and childbirth, do their
homework about hospital and doctor, and find support
with like-minded friends and midwives. Through this education, planning, and support a woman can reach that
power within herself and give birth as she chooses, as she
knows is right.

11

Emily

Premature Labor and Birth

Once again Emily was pregnant. She longed to have a second child; her son, Alex, was five years old. But Emily had trouble staying pregnant. Premature labors and deaths of several fetuses had plagued her for eight years, and Alex had barely survived his birth at thirty-two weeks. This would be her last try.

Conception was easy. The day her period was due, Emily knew she was pregnant—she began to vomit. For eight weeks Emily threw up at least three times a day, if not more. She could barely keep anything down—a little oatmeal, perhaps, or some weak tea. She had tried everything to overcome this problem with each of her pregnancies: vitamin injections, exercise, visualization, acupuncture. At various times she had been hospitalized to receive IV fluids but had always refused any medication that she felt might hurt the fetus. She knew that at twelve weeks her vomiting would disappear, only to be replaced by a voracious appetite.

But Emily's troubles were not over. At twenty weeks she would begin medication to help control premature labor and would be expected to rest continuously. No playing with Alex, no working, no sex—bed or couch until this baby became viable. From twelve to twenty weeks she played and ate to her heart's content, then settled in for the long wait.

To help combat Emily's cabin fever, her friends visited every day, bringing supper, playmates for Alex, or vacuums and dustmops. Tim, Emily's husband, was busy with his fledgling business and did not have the time to assist with the child care or housework. Sometimes Emily wondered if getting pregnant again was the right thing, but she so wanted another baby—another living child—to replace all those newborns who had died in her arms.

Emily read novels and magazines, she watched TV, and she read to Alex until she thought she'd go crazy. Once a week she won a reprieve by being driven to her obstetrician at the medical center an hour away, to have her cervix checked for signs of premature labor. Even on medication she would sometimes have enough contractions to warrant an increase in dosage, whose side effect of increased heart rate only made her more crazy.

One day Emily couldn't stand it any longer, and she got up. She did a little housework and took a short walk outside. She played with Alex and cooked supper. She no longer cared when this baby would be born. She was thirty weeks pregnant; she knew that with today's technology her baby would have a good chance of survival.

Sure enough, just after she put Alex to bed, her waters broke and her contractions came on rapidly. She called a friend to baby-sit, and she and Tim hopped in the car for a hair-raising ride to the medical center. Emily had barely arrived at the maternity ward and taken her clothes off when Ruby was born—perfect, small, and breathing.

Ruby held her own for about an hour, cuddling skin to skin with Emily. Then she developed breathing problems and joined her age mates in the intensive care nursery (ICN). Emily, who lost very little blood and did not need stitches, joined Ruby there. The sights and sounds of the

ICN did not frighten her for she had spent many a long hour there with Alex. She held Ruby's hand while she was placed on a respirator and had an IV started. Ruby responded to Emily the best she could, grasping her finger and opening her eyes now and then when Emily spoke to her.

For two weeks Emily stayed near Ruby, pumping her breasts, touching and speaking to her daughter, as Ruby developed and recovered from jaundice, was gradually weaned from the respirator, and began to take tube feedings of breast milk. Then Ruby was able to move to the nursery at the small community hospital in Emily's town. There she learned to maintain her temperature out of an isolette, gained weight, and began to breast-feed. At one month of age Ruby went home, happy and healthy at five and a half pounds.

Finally, Emily had her second child; she felt complete. When I asked her if it was all worth it— the vomiting, the bed rest, the medications, the long wait, the weeks in the ICN—she smiled and said, "Yes!"

* * *

Emily is not alone. Many women suffer miscarriages— whether at eight weeks or at twenty—and feel deep pain for the child that might have been. Some women have pregnancies complicated by severe morning sickness, premature labor, incompetent cervix, and other conditions that may bring on a premature birth: toxemia, placenta previa, diabetes, multiple fetuses.

Emily did have her share of trouble and all the pain that comes with it. While most women only have to worry about the pain of contractions and how they will handle labor, Emily also dealt with weeks of constant nausea and vomiting that made her so weak she would often faint as she threw up. On top of that, there were weeks of boring, weakening bed rest, side effects from labor-stopping medications, and the constant worry about the survival of the baby. Emily also had to deal with the pain of a nonsupportive partner and a divorce when Ruby was a year old.

How do women do it? How do they have the guts and determination to keep on when the road ahead looks fuzzy and the outcome is uncertain at best? There are reserves inside of all of us to face life's challenges. Emily took each day one at a time, each complication one at a time, and hoped for the best. Some women turn to religion and their individual idea of a Higher Power. Emily was not a religious woman, however; she turned to her friends and her own inner strength to get her through her trying times.

Only in the past forty years or so, have women lacked the support of close female friends and family members. A woman in Emily's position a hundred years ago would have been surrounded by her mother and sisters, perhaps an aunt or two, and her female cousins. Alex would have had constant companions, and Emily would not have expected so much of her husband (which might have allowed him to be more supportive, to the level he felt comfortable with). The women in Emily's neighborhood would have provided food and housecleaning services, as they automatically did for other families in need. For Emily's friends in the 1980s, helping out was important but felt like a hassle at times—it was so out of their experience.

Today women could do more to help each other through personal crises, just as some hospital staffs have begun to do more. Emily was welcome to stay at the medical center—they had a special wing for mothers of preemies. She received three meals a day and a bed as well as use of an electric breast pump—all for a nominal fee. She was nearby so that the nurses could call her if Ruby's condition changed, and she could walk down the hall to see her daughter whenever she liked. The community hospital also had a special arrangement for mothers of babies who still needed to be hospitalized; Emily had a bed and meals there, and Alex could visit his sister more frequently. The accommodations provided by the hospitals no doubt made Ruby's recovery smoother, and she was able to go home sooner.

What can we learn from Emily and Ruby's story? Patience. Trust. The importance of support of family and friends. The power of our inner strength. We can think of our problems and know that there are others who survive bigger problems. We can remember that the pain of active labor lasts a day, generally two at most. Women like Emily live with pain day after day after day, not knowing if they will survive the pain long enough for their baby to become old enough to live outside of the womb.

We can also think about this story and wonder why some women have such a hard time while others go through pregnancy and labor without even a hint of nausea, backache, heartburn, insomnia, or swollen ankles. Are we built differently? What is our perception of pain? What is our personal meaning of crisis? We can reach out to women like Emily, support them, and learn from them. We can also look inside ourselves and discover our personal strengths and weaknesses.

Pregnancy can become a time of introspection and learning for each of us as we search for our personal answers to these questions. How do I handle pain, fear, love, assistance? What do I think of my body—do I love it for whatever size, color, and age it is, or am I constantly trying to change it? Do I understand my strengths and weaknesses? Can I ask for help, or do I always have to be in control? How is my relationship with my partner? Do we trust, honor, and respect each other?

In the right atmosphere, the right place, and right time for each of us, we can discover and grow. Pregnant woman, partner, friend, or birth attendant, there is room for all of us to reach better understanding of ourselves and to grow and change. Pregnancy, birth, and parenthood are challenging and intense times, requiring us to look within, to trust ourselves and our partner, to have patience, and to work with any adversity that comes our way.

12

Kim

Vaginal Birth After Cesarean

Kim was pregnant with her second child. She lived an hour away from our birthing center and half an hour away from the major medical center where her first child had been born. She was eight months pregnant and was looking for the right place to give birth.

Her first child had been born by cesarean for CPD (cephalopelvic disproportion). In other words, a throw-away excuse from a doctor to describe a baby and a pelvis that didn't seem to fit together, the most common reason for a primary cesarean. More likely the real reason: the combination of a doctor who followed "Friedman's curve" and a woman who had labored or pushed "too long." Kim's first baby had weighed nine pounds, a lucky break for the doctor, a "reason" to confirm his diagnosis. She had become fully dilated after twelve hours of labor and had pushed for one. After "no progress"—she was in bed, on her back, attached to a fetal monitor—could that have made a difference?—surgery was performed, and her son was born.

With her second pregnancy, Kim went back to her obstetrician at the medical center. But doubts began to nag her. The more she thought, and the more she read, the more she was convinced that she had had unnecessary surgery. She wanted to avoid it a second time. When she had been unable to convince her doctor to let her try a VBAC (vaginal birth after cesarean), she started her search for a new birth attendant and a new birth place.

She had heard about our birthing center and drove over one day to check it out. After a tour and a long conversation with me, she was convinced. Here was a place where she would be encouraged to give birth vaginally; there was no routine use of a fetal monitor. She would be able to labor in any position that she chose. I gave her a list of the doctors and midwives in the area, and she left to make her calls.

I thought about Kim after she left. She was a small woman, and it seemed like a nine-pound baby was big for her. But I knew that outside appearances could be deceptive when it came to pelvic structures, and I let my fears die.

Six weeks later, when I arrived at work at 11 P.M., Kim and her husband followed me up the stairs to the birthing center. She was in very active labor, stopping several times for contractions. I changed into my scrub suit while Kim and Alan were shown to their room by the evening shift nurse. Before long the doctor wandered in, and the party was complete.

Kim showered and walked and leaned on Alan, breathing noisily with each contraction, ending each with a loud sigh. She did not look happy, and between contractions she kept saying, "Do you think I can do it?" The doctor and I did our best to assure her that she could, and soon she was fully dilated.

Then she froze. I could see the fear in her eyes. This was as far as she got last time, and then no further. I told her she didn't have to start pushing until she was ready. The baby's heartbeat was fine, all necessary emergency equipment was set up in the hallway. She fretted and cried for a while—maybe fifteen minutes—and had no contractions. I suggested that she get into the shower with Alan, try to relax, and gather her strength and courage.

I sat on the other side of the bathroom door, hearing soft moans every few minutes, some crying and conversation. After ten or fifteen minutes I heard the unmistakable sound of a woman pushing, deep grunts and low throaty moans. I stepped into the bathroom.

"Are you all right?"

"The baby's coming, I can feel it!" Her voice sounded excited and scared. She moaned with another push. She was squatting in the shower, holding onto the handrail.

"Are you comfortable in that position?"

She took a deep breath and stuck her head around the curtain.

"No, it's killing my legs."

I suggested she come out of the shower and try the toilet or the birthing stool. I left the room to give Kim and Alan some privacy while they dried off and Alan dressed. Kim came out of the bathroom naked and sat on the birthing stool next to the bed. She pushed with her next contraction and said she found the chair much more comfortable. She smiled.

"It's really coming now, isn't it?"

The doctor sat on the floor between her legs and massaged her vagina with oil while doing a brief exam. She pushed again, and we could see her perineum bulge.

"Yes, Kim, the baby's coming," the doctor told her.

I listened to the baby's heartbeat after each push; it was reassuringly steady, a strong 136 beats per minute. Kim and Alan smiled at the sound.

This went on for several minutes, pushing and listening, Kim's noises quieter and stronger. Then we could see a few tufts of hair and a wrinkled head during each push. We asked Kim where she wanted to give birth, and she chose to sit on the chair. I assembled the necessary equipment—scissors, clamp, bulb syringe, warm blankets—and Kim pushed again.

The doctor supported her perineum as the baby's head began to emerge. Alan was at Kim's side, and I joined the doctor on the floor. Slowly, slowly, slowly, the baby's head was born—first the forehead, then the eyebrows, eyes, nose, and mouth—a very slow, controlled birth. Kim took another breath and birthed the shoulders, the chest, the hips—working hard to push out every inch of her child's body.

The doctor and I looked at each other as the entire body was finally born and the baby was lifted into Kim's arms. It was one of the biggest, longest babies we had ever seen!

The cord was clamped and cut by Alan, the placenta was born in one brief push, and Kim's perineum was checked for any damage. Only a few "skid marks," as we jokingly called them—tiny superficial skin tears that did not need stitching. We helped Kim onto the bed, where she and Alan and their new son, Jacob, could relax. Kim was ecstatic, profusely thanking us and laughing and crying all at once.

"You were the one who did it, Kim, we just watched," I said as I left the room. I took the soiled instruments and blankets to be cleaned and settled down to document the birth. The doctor lingered around the nurses' station, an unusual activity—that late at night, the doctors were usually out the door as fast as they could go. He was waiting to see how much the baby weighed.

I waited until Jacob had nursed and was peaceful in his father's arms to check his vital statistics. Alan laid him on the scales: eleven and a half pounds! Everyone could hardly believe it. This was a big baby and long—nearly twenty-three inches. And to think that a doctor two years before had said that a nine-pound baby was too big for Kim's pelvis! She glowed with satisfaction.

"I did it," was all she said.

* * *

Cesarean section. Surgery or childbirth? In some cases, both. I have attended many a cesarean that felt as joyous as any vaginal birth, and some that were surrounded with tension as a woman bled profusely or a baby's heartbeat slowed more and more. And some that seemed like a doctor's convenience.

What happened to Kim the first time? Since I wasn't there, I can never be sure, but I certainly have a good idea. Kim didn't produce on schedule. She was probably nervous in the hustle-bustle routine of the medical center: medical and nursing students observing her, waiting patiently or impatiently to learn, busy labor nurses, demanding doctors, lots of machinery and rules. Kim had said her entire labor was spent in bed attached to the monitor; peeing in a bedpan; rarely changing her position; being yelled at by the doctor to push harder—verbal harassment without physical help. The doctor soon got fed up, and Kim, feeling like a failure and powerless to do anything, signed the surgical consent form.

That feeling of failure had nagged Kim for two years. According to her, it had interfered with caring for her first son, Will. She often left him crying and went off alone, crying herself. She wasn't sure she wanted to get pregnant again, and eventually did so by accident.

Determined to have things different and understanding that her feeling of failure was linked to the cesarean, Kim did a great deal of reading and educating herself. Thank goodness she had the strength to leave the doctor who would not consider her wishes and to search out a better place.

Although the doctor and I encouraged Kim in her efforts, it was Kim who did the work—it was Kim who had the inner strength—it was Kim who gave birth. We just gave her the space to take care of herself, find her inner reserves, and tap into them. We didn't scare or confuse her with technology, machinery, and orders. We stayed within the limits of safety by being near her throughout her labor, having emergency equipment set up nearby, and listening to the baby's heartbeat frequently with the Doptone—no more than we would do for any woman.

The story of Kim and Jacob has always come to me whenever I have helped a woman give birth vaginally after a previous cesarean. I would often tell the story to a woman who was having trouble pushing, telling of eleven-and-half-pound Jacob's emergence into the world after a scant forty-five minutes of pushing. It always seemed to inspire.

The determination and strength of a laboring woman have never ceased to inspire me. To see her want things to be different, to feel her trust herself, to reach down deep inside for the strength she needs to carry on. To watch her glow as she touches her baby's head as it begins to peek from her vagina, to watch her reach with open arms for her child, slippery and wet, just born. It seems cruel to me to take that opportunity away from women because of rules and impatience. A cesarean section can save the life of a woman or baby, and for that I am grateful. But to use the operation for anything less is degrading to women, denying their strength and individuality. Any woman who wants to should have the opportunity to give birth vaginally, under her own power, and with support and care from those around her.

13

Ariel

Pain or Pleasure?

It was 3 P.M., "change of shift" in nurses' lingo, when the daytime nurses tell the evening nurses the goings-on of the day. Things had been quiet, and the report was short. Then the phone rang; it was a doctor.

"Ariel French is on her way up. I'll be right along. She's six centimeters dilated; this is her fourth baby. Please get ready for the birth."

"OK," I answered, and hung up.

I told my comrades what was up: Ariel French was well-known to the staff, the woman with absolutely painless, almost undetectable labors. Her last child had been born in the parking lot.

The doctor's office was fifteen minutes away. I set up the birth supplies in the first vacant room. I also readied another set in case we needed to make a mad dash to the parking lot again.

Soon the door opened, and Ariel came down the hall. She looked barely pregnant—a petite woman with an equally petite belly.

"Hi, Ariel, what's up?"

"The doctor says I'm in labor. Who's to know? About time this baby came anyway," she answered.

I showed her to her room; she took off her clothes and put on a nightgown. The doctor walked in.

"Let's see what's happening, Ariel, if it's all right with you," he said. She nodded, lay down, and spread her legs. She was clearly at ease with her body.

I had not noticed her having any contractions -no change of expression, movement, or sound. I listened to the baby's heartbeat while the doctor sat on the bed and did the vaginal exam.

"Well, now, you're eight, Ariel. How soon are you going to have this baby? Five minutes? Ten? Fifteen?"

We all laughed, and Ariel continued to smile, reclining in bed with her legs spread. I kept my hand on her belly and, sure enough, it tightened. I timed the tightenings while we talked—they were every two minutes, lasting a minute. This woman *was* having contractions.

"Can you feel that?" I asked as her belly rose up, contracting firmly.

"Not a thing," she said.

Three contractions later her waters broke, clear fluid pouring out of her vagina and puddling on the bed.

"Here comes the baby!" she said.

Without so much as a moan or a groan, she spread her legs further apart, and I saw the bulge at her perineum. She smiled and reached down to touch the head as it began to show. The doctor supported her perineum, Ariel gave a big sigh, and the baby slipped out. She reached down for the baby—a boy—as the doctor lifted him into her arms.

"Four boys, Ariel. How do you manage?" he said.

"Maybe it'll be a girl next time," she said, as she traced the contours of her new son's face with her fingertips. The love light in her eyes clearly showed that the gender of her newborn did not matter.

A few minutes later the placenta came, and Ariel's uterus clamped down with hardly a trickle of blood. A quick check confirmed an intact perineum. I removed the wet sheets, tucked fresh ones under mother and son, picked up the tray of birthing supplies, and left the room.

I joined the doctor at the nurses' station.

"Amazing," I said. "I'll never understand why she doesn't feel anything."

"Can't say as I understand it either," said the doctor.

A few minutes later I went back to see Ariel and her baby. He was nursing happily, and Ariel was talking with her husband on the phone. Everything had happened so fast, she had forgotten to call him. Now she was chatting cheerfully and making plans for him to pick up their other children to come and visit their new brother. I checked her uterus—still firm—and laid my hand on the baby's cheek, pink and warm. Ariel smiled as she put down the phone.

"Wasn't that fun?" she said.

* * *

True or false? Being in labor = pain. Being in labor = discomfort. Being in labor = agony. Put twenty women who have given birth in one room, and you will get as many different answers. For some women labor hurts but really doesn't bother them; for others it is a trial of terror. Ariel is the only woman I've known who felt nothing. What makes the difference, and can anything be done to change it?

Many physical factors can contribute to a woman's labor pain or lack thereof. Her position, the amount of sleep she has had, the amount of food or drink she has had, if she is attached to any machinery (monitor or IV), if she has nausea or vomiting, if she is alone or has a helpful support person with her. The position of the baby can contribute to discomfort—head very low or baby turned in a posterior position (face facing toward the woman's belly instead of her back). Time of day, the number of strangers or friends in the room, the clothing she is wearing, the temperature of the room—the list is practically endless. If something is not comfortable to the laboring woman, she may have more pain until the dis-comfort is remedied.

Generally, every woman's comfort indicators will be different, but a few are universal. Procedures being done without explanation and understanding will make the woman tense and therefore more uncomfortable. Being confined to one position for a long time—most notably on her back—can become bothersome, but other positions can become uncomfortable if they are not changed frequently. The presence of certain persons—either strangers or someone that the woman is not getting along with—can make her unable to relax.

The best way to change tension-inducing factors is to listen to the woman's requests. She may want food or drink or some ice to suck on. She may be cold and want a warm shower or a blanket, or she may be hot and want to have a cold washcloth or be naked. She may want to sit or walk or lie down. She may not want her belly touched during a contraction, or she may want it rubbed. Laboring women—given the chance—are exquisitely exact and demanding when it comes to their wants and needs. I always have felt that when a woman starts ordering her assistants around, she is in good, strong labor!

Other women—who don't or can't speak up for themselves—may need to be assisted to discover the best place or position for labor. It may mean staying with a woman constantly and moving from bed to chair to shower to leaning on a friend before she finds a good position. It may mean rubbing or pressing her lower back or adding heat or cold to her head or belly before she finally responds. Too many birth attendants—nurses, usually—leave a woman alone with her husband or friend, in an unfamiliar atmosphere, full of machines, scary noises, and annoying smells—and expect them to handle it all. The nurse views her important work as tending to the monitor, proper placement of the straps, and getting a good read-out. When the woman begins to react to her pain in a more dramatic way by moaning, yelling, crying, and thrashing about, the nurse's first instinct is to offer pain medication because the monitor reading has become more important than the woman herself. And so goes the merry-go-round.

For women fortunate enough to have chosen a birth place where they feel comfortable and can get the physical things they need, there comes the challenge of reacting to the emotional stimuli that may increase their discomfort. They may be afraid for the baby's health, they may not feel ready to be a mother, or they may want to be in control and become afraid as labor sweeps them away. They may not be getting along with their mate—or their mate may have died or divorced them during the pregnancy. Perhaps a woman has internalized frightening birth stories that she heard from her mother or friends, and she may be afraid that the same things will happen to her. A woman may be afraid of pain in general, thinking that painful feelings indicate something seriously wrong that needs to be treated—a heart attack or a broken leg, for example. Or a woman may believe that breathing a certain way will make her labor painless, and when she starts feeling pain, she may start feeling angry or helpless or simply frightened that things are not going as they are "supposed" to.

Some emotional issues can be dealt with prior to labor through counseling, visualization, or meditation. Or they may have to be dealt with on the spot. An astute birth attendant will realize there is a block causing pain and may try to get the woman to speak about it openly. I have seen labors completely stop while a woman cried about a lost relationship, a deep fear of being "ripped open," or simply the fear of not having the strength to go on. A good birth attendant will give her the space to cry, to yell, to talk about it, and then will guide her back into labor, encouraging her to move past her fears and give birth.

Pain is all relative. Yes, there is discomfort associated with being in labor and giving birth. There is also discomfort with pregnancy and parenting—although maybe not to such an intense degree. As one woman said to me, "Giving birth is the most horrible *and* the most wonderful experience imaginable." It is a time to go with the feelings, to open up to the pain, to allow it to flow through you, and to make way for your child to be born. Taking one contraction at a time, giving it your full attention, and allowing it to do its work is the way to get a baby born. Finding your most safe and comfortable birth place and birth attendants, speaking up for what you need, and trusting your body's strength and knowledge are ways to give birth with the least amount of discomfort, knowing and trusting that all women are different, all labors are different, and certainly every creature that is born is different. It will hurt, yes, *and* it will be OK—because you can do it.

14

Maria, Sandy, and Teresa

Twins!

It had been a busy month for us: thirty-five births by the twentieth. That was the usual total for the entire month, and we still had several women due—including three sets of twins. At least the expected twins would be full-term. Often the birth of twins meant prematurity—usually born a month early—and the extra problems that come with early babies, like jaundice or the inability to stay warm on their own. But full-term twins were like any full-term babies—only twice as much fun—and what a time we had at our small hospital with the three sets who were born within two days!

First came Maria and her husband, Bill. The twins Maria was carrying were their first children; Maria had had a healthy pregnancy and was nearing her fortieth week of pregnancy. She was already three centimeters dilated and fully effaced (thinned out): the twins had been determined to be headfirst, and the first twin's head was settled down into her pelvis.

Maria came to us from the doctor's office; she had been having irregular contractions all night and was tired. After resting a few hours, she started to walk the halls. By 8 P.M. she was having regular contractions and was still walking.

I stayed with her, but I didn't have the extra energy of a laboring woman, and Maria's brisk walking began to tire me out.

I was glad for the tile floor when her waters broke around 10 P.M. Maria was embarrassed, as many women are, as well as just a little shocked. I brought out the mop while Bill helped her into a clean nightie and washed her legs. Maria decided not to wear a sanitary pad but dripped as she walked. Doptone in one hand and mop in the other, I followed Bill and Maria up and down that hallway all evening. Both Maria and the babies were doing well.

Soon Maria felt the urge to push, and after a vaginal exam confirmed the headfirst position of baby number one, Maria began to push. She discovered her most comfortable position was squatting with the assistance of Bill and the doctor. I had prepared everything for the birth— checked the infant resuscitation equipment, had heated beds ready for the babies if necessary, and plenty of warm blankets.

Maria continued to squat on the delivery table as baby number one was born, the cord was clamped and cut, and her son Eli was handed to her. It was five minutes to midnight. Eli was good-sized and healthy, a lusty cry emanating from his lungs. Maria and Bill laughed and held him close. I gave him an identification (ID) band so we could be sure to tell him from his sibling. After a few minutes Maria's contractions resumed, and she began to push her other baby out. As the clock hands passed over midnight, we all laughed, knowing these twins would have different birthdays. Maria pushed harder.

At ten after midnight, Eli's brother Sam was born. While Bill held Eli, Maria cradled her new son to her breast. Sam looked as healthy as Eli, and I began to pack up my resuscitation equipment. The mood in the room was joyous; the babies were fine. After a few more minutes Maria pushed out the placenta, which appeared to be two placentas joined together, and was as big. Her uterus contracted, and her bleeding was minimal. As Bill proudly held his two sons, we cleaned Maria up and settled her in bed—no tearing, no stitches.

Maria began to nurse her babies with plenty of pillows and lots of encouragement. Bill opened a bottle of champagne, and the nursing supervisor brought Maria a turkey sandwich from the kitchen. An evening's work well done was celebrated by all. Maria and her family stayed with us a couple of days—Eli and Sam always sleeping together in the same cot, arms around each other, as they had been in utero.

The next day Sandy arrived with her husband, Scott, and their three-year-old son, Ben. Sandy was thirty-eight weeks pregnant, five centimeters dilated, completely effaced, and not yet in labor. Her babies were bottom-first, with twin number one settled down into her pelvis in a frank breech position. Sandy wanted a vaginal birth, and her doctor had agreed. They had decided to induce today, since Sandy lived an hour away and her labor with Ben had been four hours long.

At 10 A.M. the doctor broke Sandy's bag of waters, and she sat on a towel in the rocking chair and rocked. Sandy was a beautiful, quiet woman with an extraordinary smile. She sat in the chair, calmly rocking, dressed in a soft, lilac flannel nightgown as the contractions began. She never made a sound as the contractions increased in strength and length, just concentrated on a spot on the far wall and rocked. I could tell when a contraction was over because she would turn to me and smile.

After an hour Sandy got up for a brief shower and returned to sit, naked, on the small birthing stool. She continued her pattern of concentrating and smiling; I listened to the babies' heartbeats, which were fine, as Scott and Ben sat on the bed and quietly read books.

When Sandy started to push, we readied all the emergency equipment and gathered the necessary nurses and doctors for the birth. Sandy settled herself onto the delivery table in a semi-squat, without the stirrups. She continued to look angelic, with only a few drops of perspiration appearing on her face. She pushed gently but firmly, and soon bottom number one appeared—it was a boy! After Jason's bottom was born, his legs popped out, the doctor's hands guided the body and head out, and Jason took his first breath. It was just noon.

Sandy held Jason while Scott and Ben looked on, and we waited for baby number two to start its descent. The doctor confirmed another breech position—feet first—and soon a set of toes was wiggling in the warm air of the room. Sandy pushed again with the same quiet determination and baby number two slowly emerged—feet, legs, bottom, torso, arms, and head—a girl! Ashley appeared as gracefully as Jason had, slipping out of her mother's vagina without fuss, and joined her brother at Sandy's breast.

Again the mood in the room was joyous—another twin birth, and breech at that, completed without complications. Problems can crop up at any time, and the added factors of twins and breech made us all the more nervous and prepared, yet here were two lovely plump babies contentedly nursing. Sandy held her serene mood through the birth of the placenta and a check of her vagina and perineum. Again, no stitches necessary.

After settling Sandy and Scott and their newly expanded family in their room, we cleaned up the delivery room in anticipation of the third set of twins—things always seemed to come in threes. Would the third set come soon, and would that labor and birth be equally uneventful?

By midnight we had found out. Teresa and Todd had arrived after laboring most of the day at home. Now Teresa was starting to push. Her twins were her first children—

twin number one was headfirst, and number two was breech—and they were healthy and strong. When the first baby's head began to show a little during a push, Teresa and Todd walked to the delivery room, where things were set up.

Slowly, slowly, twin number one's head emerged with gentle and controlled pushing on Teresa's part. The head was born, the shoulders slipped out easily, and Teresa reached down for her daughter as the body was born. Jennifer cried and was covered with warm blankets while Teresa held her. Another easy birth, another healthy baby.

After giving Teresa a few minutes to enjoy her newborn, the doctor checked the position of twin number two. Unfortunately, the baby was no longer breech but had slipped into a transverse, or sideways, position after its sibling had been born. A shoulder seemed to be caught in Teresa's cervix. Twin number two's heartbeat had always been steady and strong and continued to be, so the two doctors present attempted to push the shoulder up and birth the baby in a feet-first breech position. But this baby was too well settled in, and after an hour of attempts to change its position, it was clearly time for another solution.

The problem was discussed with Teresa and Todd, and they decided on a cesarean. The operating room was set up, and they signed the permit for surgery. Jennifer was left in the care of a nurse, and the rest of the birthing crew headed for the operating room.

The mood was light as the time drew closer to 3 A.M. Teresa's belly was prepped—pubic hair shaved, abdomen washed with an antiseptic solution, and a urinary catheter inserted—after she had received spinal anesthesia. The surgeon began his work as everyone waited in anticipation. Three minutes later Jessica was born, as sturdy and as healthy as her sister.

Todd and Jessica returned to their room to be reunited with Jennifer while Teresa finished with surgery. Father and daughters cuddled happily in bed, wrapped well with warm blankets. Teresa's belly and the small tear on her perineum were stitched up. She had experienced two contrasting births in one night's hard work, and spent the next four days recovering from both and learning how to care for her babies.

Maria, Teresa, and Sandy enjoyed each other's company over the next few days as they adjusted to their newly expanded families. The men enjoyed the presence of the other men going through the same feelings of delight, fear, and awe. We had fun watching the babies nestled together with their parents, thankful that all six were good-sized and healthy.

*   *   *

Twins. Double the fun or double the trouble? Carrying two or more babies is a challenging task for any woman. Maria, Teresa, and Sandy had easier pregnancies than many. Some women are plagued with swollen ankles, varicose veins, and high blood pressure, and spend most of their pregnancy lying down. One woman I knew had invested in a waterbed, the only place she could be comfortable and relaxed. These three women were pleased that their babies had been full-term; many twins come early because they slowly run out of space.

But twins are definitely more work—more diapers, more feedings, less sleep. Even the strongest women can have a hard time coping for the first few months. Although two babies can cause more trouble—certainly once they are born—they do not necessarily mean more trouble during labor and birth. Most physicians classify multiple pregnancies as high-risk and do not let women have the labor and birth they choose but instead pull out all the high-tech stops for a doctor-orchestrated birth. This is not necessary, especially for twins.

Although at the time of these twins' births we had a policy that they be born in the delivery room, as time went on, twin births began to take place in bed instead of on the delivery table. But even in the delivery room all was casual. The women were encouraged to squat when they were pushing and to climb up on the table only at the time of birth. We thought of the table as no more than a small and unusual bed. The stirrups and forceps were there in case of complications only.

The physical appearance of a birth place matters less than many people think. Delicately flowered wallpaper, matching curtains, and oak furniture are certainly attractive, but it is the atmosphere and attitude that count the most. Even in the most lovely places, if the birth attendants have their own agendas and ignore the needs and wants of the woman, the physical beauty matters little. I have been at births in cars, in hallways, in bathrooms, in rooms no bigger than closets and just as dark, and in each instance the place mattered little. What mattered was that the woman gave birth as she chose, reaching down for her child as it was born, surrounded by people she loved.

In an atmosphere of mistrust and medicalized routine, Maria, Teresa, and Sandy would have had very different experiences. At the very least, they all would have been attached to fetal monitors during their entire labor. And probably only Maria would have been allowed to labor. Sandy, with her two breech babies, would have had an automatic cesarean and Teresa, with one breech baby, would most likely have had a cesarean as well. Many doctors are frightened of vaginal breech births—frightened of complications that could lead to lawsuits. And sad to say, as time goes on, there are fewer and fewer birth attendants who even know *how* to help a breech baby be born. The skill is rarely taught anymore as the cesarean-for-breech policy becomes almost universal in this country.

But in an atmosphere of "watch and wait," with well trained and respectful nurses and doctors, these three women labored the best way they knew how and gave birth as their body required. We were there, during labor and birth, assisting the women and their partners through this crucial time. In a situation that would have been considered high-risk anywhere else, we were ready to do what was necessary to help these mothers and babies pass through their birth journey safely. We never lost sight of the woman-centered process.

Their postpartum experiences were different as well. Except for the time Teresa was in the OR, each set of twins was always close to their mother and to each other—if not in the same bed. Most other hospitals would have required a stay in the nursery and separate beds. We knew the importance of keeping these babies together—why further disrupt what they have known so well for nine months? Even sick twins who needed some close observation in the special nursery stayed together in the same isolette. I expect it calmed the babies and allowed them to heal faster.

By giving the mothers, fathers, and babies the time and private space to be together, they learn faster and feel more comfortable with what comes next. Keeping babies separated from their parents helps no one but the nursing staff. Newborns crave contact, warmth, and closeness. Beginning life in the motionless, unnaturally quiet, and bright atmosphere of an isolette must be torture for a baby who has known only darkness, wet warmth, gentle motion, and the voices of his or her family. Birth attendants must remember that the parents and child(ren) are a unit not to be disturbed by routine hospital procedures.

Twin births are special; I remember each one that I have attended, and feel honored and amazed by them all. To think that *two* babies grew and developed together, always in contact and aware of each other. To see them emerge, one after the other, to begin the next phase of their life together, is always moving. I am grateful for the opportunity to have participated in peaceful and family-centered births with all of them.

15

Elaine and Janet

Meconium Aspiration and Shoulder Dystocia

I had barely hung up the phone with the admitting desk clerk when two women came hurrying down the hall. The pregnant one was slender and tall; her companion, short and round. The tall woman leaned on the short one as another contraction engulfed her. I approached them, waited for the contraction to end, and showed them to their room. Elaine, the pregnant one, had two contractions before we could get there. She was making grunting noises at the peak of the contraction—things were moving right along.

We entered the room at the end of the hall, a bright and sunny space with two large windows. Pam helped Elaine take off her pants and underwear, leaving her big T-shirt on. I started to ask them about the labor—when it had started, how far apart the contractions were—when I decided it was useless information. This baby was clearly getting born soon. I listened to the baby's heartbeat—it sounded fine, around 120. Elaine said she had to pee, and I showed her to the bathroom.

I was talking to Pam, giving her a brief verbal tour of the unit—the kitchen, the linens, the nurses' station—when a yell came from the bathroom.

"Help! What's this!"

Pam and I rushed in, and Elaine held up a piece of toilet paper. It was covered with a dark green stain. Meconium. Thick. Fresh.

"Where did that come from Elaine? Your vagina?" She nodded.

She stood up, and the gooey substance began moving down her inner thighs, slowly, stickily.

I listened to the baby's heartbeat: 112. Elaine had another contraction, said she felt pressure, had to push. I was on the phone in an instant. The doctor would be there shortly. I rang the nurse's call bell and another nurse arrived.

"Call the pediatrician. Get the resuscitation stuff set up. Meconium. Thick."

There was in me both a sense of panic and a sense of calm. I looked at Elaine and Pam's frightened faces and tried to explain what was happening. The doctor walked in. Elaine had a contraction and involuntarily pushed. I listened to the baby—the heartbeat was erratic, running between 100 and 120, finally settling at 120.

The doctor and I got Elaine on the bed. A vaginal exam confirmed a baby on the way down the birth canal and gobs of fresh meconium.

Meconium—a baby's first bowel movement, released under stress. Fine to do on the outside, but when on the inside, a grave danger. One deep breath of the sticky, tarry substance and a baby becomes severely ill. Imagine trying to breathe with that stuff coated on the inside of the lungs. Plenty of work cut out for the birth attendants—get that stuff suctioned out of the baby's mouth, nose, and throat as soon as possible, before the baby can take a breath. Clear it out. Make way for life-giving oxygen.

The doctor was explaining the situation to Pam and Elaine as I set up the heated bed, laryngoscope, tubes, sterile water, syringes, Delee suction sets, ambu bag, oxygen. The doctor explained the equipment and the process—Elaine should push steadily and easily, and be ready to stop on command. The pediatrician and another nurse arrived.

One nurse was listening to the baby constantly now as I readied the resuscitation equipment, checking once more that everything was there and accessible. We worked with an unspoken rhythm—she would stay with Elaine and Pam and help with the birth and placenta, I would work with the pediatrician and baby. The thump-thump-thump of the heartbeat echoed throughout the room, the thumps slowing with each push and then gradually returning to 120 beats per minute. Pam held the oxygen mask, and Elaine breathed deeply between each contraction as she nestled her head on Pam's shoulder.

We could see the head now, covered with the dangerous goo, slowly emerging. Elaine was doing a great job pushing evenly, steadily. Then the head was out and the pediatrician suctioned the mouth and nose with a Delee. Worthless; the stuff was too thick.

"Push. Now." the doctor said, and the baby slithered out into his hands. He hastily clamped and cut the cord, stepped to the end of the bed, and placed the baby in the heated bed.

The baby was limp, blue, a faint pulse at the base of the cord where it joined the baby's body. The pediatrician had already begun to intubate and suck the meconium out as fast as possible. Laryngoscope into the throat, tube inserted, syringe of water squirted in, suck. We repeated the process over and over. I drew up syringes of water as fast as I could and handed them to the pediatrician along with new tubes. Insert, water, suck. One minute gone by, then two.

The baby, a boy, still had a pulse, but it was weakening. Time to let him breathe. The last suck had brought up a thinner, paler substance. Time to stimulate. I rubbed the soles of his feet, his back, spoke to him. The pediatrician held the ambu bag over his face, ready to breathe for him. David took a breath, spluttered, blinked. Come on baby, do it again, do it again! David took another breath and another. His heartbeat increased; soon it was 120. Three minutes had gone by.

The pediatrician and I stood over David and watched his color change from purple to pink. His breaths came in gasps, but he breathed—on his own. By five minutes of age his gasping had calmed, and he was breathing regularly but rapidly. I looked over at Elaine and Pam and smiled.

"He's doing O.K., he's breathing."

They held each other and sobbed. It had all happened so fast—they had been in the hospital barely twenty minutes. While I held the oxygen near David's face, the pediatrician spoke to the women. He explained about meconium aspiration and the seriousness of the possible consequent pneumonia. He said David would need to go to an intensive care nursery (ICN) where he could be watched and cared for with equipment more sophisticated than ours. He gave them a choice of two hospitals, they chose the one closer to their home, and we put the transfer process in motion.

I took David to the special nursery and stayed with him. I put him in an isolette, hooked up the oxygen, and comforted him the best I could while checking his vital signs and preparing for blood tests. A few minutes later the pediatrician arrived, and then the other nurse. She reported that the placenta had arrived without incident, and Elaine had received a couple of stitches to a small perineal tear. Pam and Elaine wanted to know if they could see David.

While the pediatrician made the call to the ICN, Pam helped Elaine to the nursery. I showed them how to put their hands through the portholes to touch their son. Each woman reached in to touch David and held each other with her free arm. I stayed nearby watching David's color and breathing but far enough away to give them a sense of privacy. They began to ask me questions, and I moved closer to answer. They told me of their struggle to have David—convincing the local infertility clinic to give them artificial insemination, dealing with homophobia, then the endless tries, temperature taking, mucus checks, mad dashes to the clinic. It took six months before Elaine became pregnant. The pregnancy was healthy and happy, and they looked forward to the baby who would complete their family. And here he was, under plastic, eyes closed, concentrating only on each rapid, shallow breath, trying to stay alive.

Within an hour the transport team had arrived and readied David for his trip to the medical center. Elaine and Pam packed up to leave, to follow David to the ICN and stay with him there. Soon everyone was gone, and after a half hour's cleanup there were no traces of the two women and their new son. Only the memory of a close call and a resuscitation well done.

The next day I was checking the resuscitation equipment with another nurse when Janet showed up in early labor. She was pregnant with her third child and had been dropped off by her husband. He did not want to be at the birth but would stay home to take care of the other kids. Janet didn't seem concerned, she'd been through this before. I walked her to her room, where she undressed and decided to have a shower. I returned to the equipment check.

Twenty minutes later Janet wandered down the hall. She said her contractions were irregular—seven to ten minutes apart—but she knew things would be fast once they got going. I listened to the baby's heartbeat; it sounded fine. Janet sat in a chair at the nurses' station.

The three of us chatted—it was a quiet morning without much else to do. Janet got some juice from the kitchen and

walked around a bit. Then she quietly stuck her head in
the door and said she'd made a mess—her waters had broken down the hall. The other nurse got the mop, and I listened to the baby's heartbeat. It was still fine. Janet and I
walked up the hall to her room, where she put on a sanitary pad and belt to catch the drips.

"Won't be long," she said.

The other nurse and I looked at each other with curiosity. The contractions still were irregular, but Janet seemed
to know what was going on.

Sure enough, about five minutes later, they hit—long,
strong contractions, two minutes apart. We started to
ready things for the birth.

Janet paced the floor, going from windowsill to windowsill, leaning on them during each contraction. Previously
silent during contractions, she now began to make noise,
softly at first, then louder and louder. She had an odd
combination of moans and deep breaths, hardly relaxed,
but with a quiet determination on her face. She was working hard. Windowsill to windowsill, breathe moan breathe
moan. The other nurse stayed with Janet while I called the
doctor.

As soon as I got off the phone, Janet started making
pushing noises. She climbed onto the bed, gathered herself into a semi-squat and started to bear down. Here was
a woman who knew what she was doing—never been to a
childbirth class, no support from her husband, but she
knew how to have babies. The other nurse listened to the
heartbeat as I rechecked the birthing supplies. Everything
was ready.

Two contractions later, the head appeared and slowly
emerged. I reached out my hands to support the perineum as the doctor walked into the room. The head was
born by the time he stepped up to the bed. The baby grim-
aced, and we all laughed. Then Janet squealed—the baby
had kicked. We laughed again and told her to push to get
the little troublemaker out.

Janet pushed and pushed. Nothing. Just a head getting more purple by the second.

"Harder, Janet, give it all you've got," said the doctor. No movement. We encouraged her again. Nothing.

"Get her on her hands and knees. Call the pediatrician. Get the heated bed in here," the doctor barked. We knew what was happening and, again, worked in a smooth rhythm—the other nurse helped with Janet while I made the phone call and moved the equipment into the room.

I returned to the room in time to see the doctor reaching past the baby's head into Janet's vagina. I knew what he was doing and it worked—he had reached in for the baby's arm, swung it around, and "corkscrewed" the baby out.

The other nurse clamped and cut the cord, and the doctor placed the baby, a girl, in the heated bed. The baby had no pulse, and I began chest compressions while the doctor placed the ambu bag over the baby's face and started breathing for her. The other nurse stayed with Janet, and out of the corner of my eye I watched her slip the placenta into a basin and massage Janet's uterus.

"She's bleeding too much," I heard her say.

"Give her some Pitocin," said the doctor, and I watched the nurse draw the drug up into a syringe and inject it into Janet's thigh.

By now the baby's heart was beating on its own. I watched her blink her eyes and take a breath. She struggled for another breath and then another, and soon she was breathing on her own. The pediatrician walked in. It had been five minutes since Becky had been born.

The mood changed, calmness replacing frantic activity. The pediatrician checked out Becky, the doctor kept a hand on Janet's uterus. The other nurse and I looked at each other and smiled. I could see her holding Janet's hand and softly explaining to her what had happened.

After ten minutes Becky no longer needed oxygen. There did not seem to be any broken bones, but the pediatrician wanted to do some X rays to make sure. I wheeled the heated bed over to Janet. As Janet reached for Becky's hand, a big tear rolled down her cheek. After her great noises of labor, Janet had returned to her quiet, shy self.

Becky went to the nursery for X rays, and Janet had a few stitches for a small tear. She was lucky not to have torn more with Becky's violent birth. She was weak from her heavy bleeding and remained in bed. When Becky's X rays were done—no broken bones—we returned her to her mother. Another miracle. Less than an hour before, Becky had been limp and purple with no sign of life. Yet here she was—pink and wide awake, gazing at her mother. We left them alone together.

                              *   *   *

Meconium aspiration and shoulder dystocia. Two of the most frightening birth complications.

Meconium aspiration. The number one killer of otherwise healthy, full-term babies. A complication that may show up at the last second and one that only well-trained birth attendants can handle. A classic reason for a home-to-hospital transfer. A scary situation for those who attend home births—and almost as scary for those in a well-equipped hospital. Even more frightening for the parents.

David, Elaine, and Pam were lucky. David spent ten days in the ICN and went home a happy, healthy baby. They were supported all along the way—at both the community hospital and the ICN. We tried to lessen their fear by explaining the situation, the equipment, what would happen. We gave them the space to be with their child. We hid nothing from them—the resuscitation happened at the foot of their bed, and they came to the nursery to be with David as soon as they could. They left, less than two hours after the birth, to be with their son.

There is no predicting which baby will pass meconium so close to birth time, and no one will ever really know why. Yes, "overdue" babies tend to come meconium-stained more often than other babies, but that is no guarantee. A baby with certain physical deformities or a poorly functioning placenta may pass meconium. But, more commonly, meconium shows up as a pale yellow-green tint to otherwise clear fluid—it could have been there for days or even weeks—and does not pose as great a risk. Just another mystery in the dance of birth.

Same with shoulder dystocia. A doctor or midwife may try to predict the size of the baby and do so with fair accuracy, but "stuck" shoulders happen when the size of the baby and the size of the woman's pelvic structure do not fit well. And that cannot always be predicted—just handled when it happens. All the birth attendant can do is try to "spring" the shoulders from the pelvic outlet, even if she or he has to break an arm or a collarbone in the process. Better to be out—broken bones can heal. Becky was lucky to be born without broken bones, but it would not have been unusual in her situation. She was lucky to be alive and not have any aftereffects from her birth.

These complications are serious, and in the rush to save the baby the parents may be forgotten. Ignorance of the situation increases their anxiety—they've just been through the intensity of pregnancy and labor, expecting to rejoice in the birth of their child, to hold the baby close in their arms and gaze upon the curious little face, marveling at toes and fingers, Grandpa's nose, and Aunt Ethel's ears. All that hard work and *whoosh!* the baby is gone. Did they dream it all? In some places they may not see their child for days, feeling bereft and unable to believe the child is really theirs when they finally see the baby.

Even in the rush and tension of preparation, with the unusual equipment and hurrying people, someone can be there with the parents, explaining what is happening and why. If all the birth attendants know their roles and work well together, someone will take a place at the side of the mother, focusing on her and her partner. Maybe simply holding her hand, expressing calm with touch. Giving them information as they are ready. Doing everything possible to help the parents be with their child, even if it means leaving the birth place so soon. If the mother is unable to go, her partner or a friend or relative can accompany the baby. Bringing the baby, in the isolette or heated bed, to the mother. With portable oxygen, equipment on wheels, and plenty of electrical outlets there should be no problem. A nurse can observe the baby in the mother's room as well as in the nursery.

It is important for birth attendants to take steps to ensure the life of the mother and child. It is also important to remember where that child came from, and why. That child emerged from a woman's body—the mother—and that's where the child belongs: with her and with her partner. Those are the family members. A child has been born to a family and not to the hospital staff. Although people come to hospitals with the intention of being cared for, the integrity of the family must be maintained at the same time the care is given. It can be done without sacrificing safety or costing a fortune.

Giving birth is more than a physical act with physical needs that have to be met: blood soaked up with pads, perineum to be cleaned, uterine tone to be felt, vital signs to be taken, food and drink to be offered. Giving birth is a deeply emotional and psychological event. More than anything, the family needs to be together—as they have been for the last nine months. Complicated or routine, each birth, each family, needs to be respected for its choices, its needs, and its love.

16

Rebecca

Teen Mom

I befriended Rebecca in her fourth month of pregnancy. Seventeen years old, alone, living in desperate poverty in an abandoned school bus with no electricity or running water, she was happy to have a friend. Rebecca's parents had thrown her out of the house when she turned fifteen, and she dropped out of school in the middle of her sophomore year. Moving from relatives to friends, supporting herself as a checkout girl in a grocery store, she found herself pregnant and abandoned by her boyfriend.

Rebecca lived a backwoods life, five miles up a dirt road, on the land of an old mountain patriarch, a family friend. Several shacks and abandoned vehicles provided shelter for the residents, who changed frequently. I took Rebecca shopping, to the thrift shop, to doctor's appointments, and to childbirth classes. I loaned her pregnancy and childbirth books that she read voraciously along with the *National Enquirer* and *Star Magazine*. She was intelligent and understood it all.

Her pregnancy was a birth control failure: foam. At least she had tried. But she had accepted the pregnancy as a guarantee that she would finally have a family and someone to love. She wanted to have the baby naturally and planned to breast-feed. At the time, I was a nursing mother of a six-month-old who came with us on all our trips.

Rebecca's pregnancy was uneventful. My biggest challenge was to dispel the old wives' tales that she heard from other women. Tales about "marked" babies, and dry births, and certain activities making the cord be around the neck, breast-feeding making you unattractive, and the awful things that visiting nurses could do to you. Rebecca wanted to do everything the best way possible. Her questions included "What are the best hot dogs to eat during pregnancy?" I visited her as a friend, not as a nurse, but she knew my background and pressed me for answers. I hated to tell her hot dogs were not good at all, knowing she had to survive on welfare and food stamps.

On a cold night in December, she called me in tears, saying she had been having pains every seven minutes all day and that the nurse at the doctor's office told her she wasn't really in labor. Rebecca was at the home of an extended family member who was pumping her full of hospital and doctor horror stories, and she was scared. I went right over.

I sat with Rebecca and calmed her down, offering her juice to drink and a cool cloth for her forehead. Her contractions were now five minutes apart and, although mild, were quite regular. After a couple of hours she asked to go to the hospital.

The local hospital was small and friendly, and the maternity ward was quiet that night. It was midnight by the time we arrived and settled in. Rebecca was four centimeters dilated. The nurse left us alone. Rebecca and I dozed in between contractions for a couple of hours until she cried out.

"It really hurts, I don't know what to do!"

I got up and helped her into the shower, and we stayed in the bathroom for the next few hours. The nurse checked in periodically to listen to the baby's heartbeat and to see how we were doing. I sat on the toilet and encouraged Rebecca every time she called out for me. The contractions were three minutes apart when we moved back to the birthing room and the nurse checked her—eight centimeters. Rebecca was thrilled that she had progressed so far—and without drugs.

Then the vomiting began. Rebecca threw up or retched with every contraction. The labor became a burden to her. She began to cry, and no amount of coaxing or cajoling or encouraging her could stop the vomiting or the tears. The nurse offered her some Vistaril, which might help stop the vomiting.

Rebecca was worried that by taking this drug she would be a "failure" or would hurt the baby in some way. I told her that it would be a small amount that would mostly help the vomiting, and it wouldn't hurt the baby. She had the shot. An hour later she was fully dilated and began to push. The vomiting had stopped.

Rebecca got herself comfortable in a semi-squat in bed and pushed with each contraction. She got more and more excited as the baby got closer to being born. She reached down and touched the baby's head as it began to emerge. With encouragement and quiet guidance she pushed the baby's head out slowly and gently, and did not tear. The doctor placed the baby on her belly. It was a girl. The placenta came easily, and Rebecca put her daughter to her breast. Amelia was a natural and took to nursing right away. The doctor and nurse left the three of us alone together.

It was strange for me to be in the partner role instead of the nurse role, but I relished every moment. I helped Rebecca make phone calls to her sisters and her mother. I held Amelia while Rebecca had a shower and the nurses cleaned up. That evening I returned to share a special dinner with Rebecca and Amelia: this hospital offered a formal dinner to all new parents, complete with menu, white tablecloth, and sparkling nonalcoholic wine. I had often thought such gimmicks were a bit "hokey," but for Rebecca, who had never been out to dinner in her life, it was a dream come true.

Rebecca and Amelia did well after the birth. Breast-feeding went well, and when Amelia was six months old, Rebecca moved to the city and got her own apartment and a job. She was determined that Amelia would have a different life than she had had—a mother who cared and worked and was not on welfare. Rebecca's dream materialized for a few months; then Amelia's father showed up, and Rebecca gave birth to her son Charles, nine months later. The American dream dies hard: Rebecca had been pulled into the coupledom and parenthood that is a sign of maturity and success in our culture.

I have kept in touch with Rebecca. Charles's and Amelia's father continues to be unemployed and Rebecca does it all—earning money, child care, housework—but she is happy and feels strong. She is out of the welfare system and is working hard to provide a good life for her family. My only wish for her is a participating partner. I know she has the power to carry on and, most important, so does she.

*   *   *

I present Rebecca's story for several reasons: to illustrate the importance of supportive birth attendants, and of choosing the right birth place, and to show that even "ignorant" young women can give birth without excessive intervention. I have experienced the attitude of many doctors and nurses time and time again: if a woman doesn't specifically request certain things—no sedation, no episiotomy, no IV, for example—she will be treated according to the "rules," in a cattle-herding, nonempowering way.

When the birthing rooms were first conceived at one hospital where I worked, they were available only for women who had attended classes, had a partner, and wanted a "certain experience." Sue Smith, who lived down the road and had another baby every year, did not count. She was relegated to a labor room and a "sterile" birth in a delivery room. Time soon changed this policy.

All women used the birthing room, young or old, prepared or unprepared, high-risk or low-risk. They all labored with a minimum of intervention and just the right amount of monitoring—by a nurse, not a machine. They all gave birth in the room, in bed or squatting on the floor; no one had an episiotomy unless she needed it; and all babies roomed-in unless they were sick and required special care. The women who were the most empowered and thrilled by their experience were the ones least prepared for it. They would repeat over and over to friends and relatives that they gave birth right there in the bed, they had no drugs, they had no stitches, and best of all, the baby was right there beside them! I often wondered how much child abuse was being prevented and how many women were just beginning to discover the power they had to change their lives in other ways.

When a woman gives birth consciously and with awareness among people who respect every woman's power, the experience can be enough to transform her life. Rebecca spoke to me after Charles's birth and said how disappointed she was because it had been so long and hard. She had had no support person with her because the baby's father didn't believe in such a thing, and she had no women friends or relatives she could trust. She was alone, without the encouragement and support she had had for Amelia's birth.

No matter a woman's social class, educational level, age, and marital status, she is still a woman giving birth who needs special attention and care. She needs at least one caring loved one with her to help ease her way. There are many women in your community who are giving birth alone, without partners or friends, for many reasons. You can help support them, or ask for support for yourself, by contacting your local childbirth educators, midwives, or visiting nurses. They can pair up women who need each other. My experience with Rebecca was very special, an enlightening experience for both of us, and one that may yet transform Rebecca's life. I believe a little voice will always be with her saying, "If I had the strength to give birth to my child, I can do anything."

17

Linda

Birth Among Family and Friends

On cue, Linda's waters broke. Pregnant with her fourth child, she had wondered how this labor would begin. She was nearly an hour from the hospital and wanted plenty of warning because her previous labors had been fast. Her six-year-old daughter, Opal, had been born after four hours of labor that started six hours after her waters broke. Two years later, with twins Rick and Jim, the same scenario had repeated itself—only shorter. She had leapt out of bed at four on that winter morning, only to have clear fluid drench her bedroom floor. By 5:30 A.M. they were at the hospital, and just after 7 A.M. her sons were born, one after the other as she squatted on the delivery room table.

It was nearly eleven that night as Linda mopped up the fluid from her bathroom floor. Fred was getting the kids up and dressed. Linda called her mother and her midwife, and then they were on their way. By the time they reached the hospital, it was nearing midnight, and Linda was having a few mild contractions.

Her mother and the midwife were already there in the only room available. The family piled in, sleepy and excited, kids heading for the big chair in the corner and

Grandma's lap. Linda was laughing and Fred was busy with the bags—books, crayons, and paper for the kids, a few things for Linda. I was to have the pleasure of being at this birth as a friend and not as a nurse.

The room was full of people: besides Linda and her family, Grandma, myself, and the midwife, there were the two regular on-duty nurses—ten people in all. Linda was not afraid of crowds, and besides, we were all friends. It was nearly the same group that had assembled for the births of Rick and Jim four years previously, with the addition, at that time, of a couple of doctors. To top it all off, the midwife was nine months pregnant—it had been a toss-up all along who would give birth first.

As Linda's contractions grew stronger, she and Fred slipped into a comfortable rhythm. With each contraction Linda would lean on the bedside table and slowly rock her hips. Fred would press on her lower back and move with her. The room would fall silent as they worked with each contraction, Linda never making a sound, not breathing in any noticeable way, simply moving in time with an inner beat. Contraction over, Linda would stand up and continue the conversation where it had left off.

The kids cuddled with Grandma in the corner. They did not appear afraid, just tired and excited. Opal had been at her brothers' birth, but she could not really remember the event. Linda and Fred had prepared them well—they had attended several prenatal visits and had seen a birth movie. This was a family that spent a great deal of time together, and the children were always well-prepared for any occasion.

After an hour or so Linda decided to take a shower. She and Fred disappeared into the bathroom and hopped into the shower together. They continued their rocking and pressure duet to the beat of the water on Linda's back. Twenty minutes later Linda emerged and said, "It's time to push!"

She positioned herself in a semi-squat on the bed while the midwife checked her—fully dilated and ready to go. After trying a push on the bed, Linda moved to the floor, where, holding onto Fred, she could assume a full squat. We waited as Linda gave several solid pushes, a low moan coming from deep in her throat.

All of a sudden, as the baby's head neared the opening, Linda asked to be in the bed. She could not walk with all the pressure, so Fred and I, on either side, carried her to the bed. There she automatically reached down to her vulva and touched the slowly emerging head. Together, the midwife and Linda guided the baby's head out, and Linda reached down and lifted her third son onto her belly.

The kids, who had been waiting on Grandma's lap, suddenly made a rush for the bed. Instantly they were at their mother's side, and the rest of us stepped back so they could greet their new brother. It was a small bed, but they all managed to get on. No one even noticed when the placenta came a few minutes later, and after inspecting Linda's intact perineum and checking her firm uterus, we left the family alone.

When I returned to the room a bit later, Opal, Rick, and Jim were taking turns holding their brother Cedar. Grandma and Dad were assisting the kids, while Linda was in the shower, cleaning up. I changed the sheets on the bed and straightened up the room. Linda returned to bed, refreshed and clean, and nursed her new son. Grandma packed up the kids, and they left to spend the rest of the night at her house. Fred got into bed with Linda and Cedar, and they settled down for sleep.

In the morning when I returned to the hospital—this time to work—Linda and Fred were getting ready to go home. I was sorry my friend was leaving so soon, but I could understand her desire to be in her own bed and eat her own food. I knew she was in good hands—her mother

and Fred had cared for her well after Opal, Rick, and Jim
had been born, and this time would be no different. I held
Cedar briefly as his parents packed up, and I looked upon
his peaceful face. What a lucky boy to have joined such a
loving family!

*   *   *

Ah, if they could all be so simple! Linda never appeared
to be in pain. She had no need of any breathing patterns
or other distractions. She knew her body, she felt at home
with her power, and she was happy to work with her
uterus and cervix as they opened for Cedar's exit. She was
surrounded by her entire family and the friends who
meant the most to her. Her mother was there, a calming
presence. She trusted herself, her attendants, her place.

So why aren't they all like this? Because, as with body
type, eye color, and personality, we are all different. No
one wants every person to look the same and be the
same—life would be altogether too boring! The same holds
true with birth. Certain events are guaranteed—at some
point the waters break, at some point there are contractions, at some point the baby is pushed out, the vagina ex-
pands, and the vulva stretches to accommodate the child.
The baby eventually comes out, grimaces, opens its eyes,
breathes, cries. The cord stops pulsing and the placenta
comes out. The uterus contracts, its work done. If any of
these events doesn't happen, there are ways to help. An
amnihook or a fingernail can release the waters; lovemaking, herbs, castor oil, acupuncture, or Pitocin can stimulate contractions; forceps, vacuum extraction, or surgery
can help a baby out. An episiotomy can open a perineum
that does not yield. Stimulation, oxygen, an ambu bag, or
CPR can help a baby start to breathe and come alive. A
hand reached into the uterus or surgery can help a placenta that refuses to budge, and breast stimulation, herbs,
Pitocin, or ice or massage to the uterus can help a boggy
womb firm up and staunch the flow of blood.

Some birth attendants do not trust the natural process and use some or all of these aids as a routine, without giving the body time to handle things on its own. I prefer to let nature take her course and think of these interventions as just that—ways to intervene if things do not happen on their own with simple help and encouragement. Childbirth is full of technology—clearly unnecessary in Linda's case—technology that needs to be used as a last-ditch attempt. "Appropriate" technology, if you will.

More than once, I have been very thankful for oxygen and Pitocin and a nearby operating room. I have watched babies come back to life and women nearly bleed to death. It can happen. It does happen—but rarely.

Most births are like Linda's, with slight variations—length of labor, length of pushing time, ways that women handle contractions, the sounds or lack of sounds, the help or hindrance of partners, the types of positions, the preference for showers or pacing the floor. These are as individual as the individual woman. There is no right or wrong. There is no one way. When a woman sets herself up with a "right"/"wrong" dichotomy, problems begin.

For one woman, the "right" way may be silence because she thinks noise only comes with "lack of control." For another, "right" means a birth at home and never, under any circumstances, in the hospital. For a third, she must not feel pain—any pain. For a fourth, she must squat to give birth even though it is uncomfortable for her. I could go on and on. In childbirth classes, people ask me over and over, "Just exactly how should I breathe?" Or, "Just how long is labor?" They are very frustrated when my answers do not provide them with anything more than "averages" and "This is what happens to *some* people."

But a few can accept the "unknown" aspect of childbirth. Some people are not fazed by what might or might not happen. They know that whatever comes their way will be all right and that they can handle it. They have thought through their choices—the aspects of the process that they can control: birth attendant, birth place, whether they want pain medication or an IV or a fetal monitor or an episiotomy or breast-feeding. They make written birth plans if necessary: they are organized in their thoughts. They bring a friend to help speak for them if the going gets rough. They are prepared.

Not "prepared" in a way that means they practiced their breathing diligently every day for three months or did their perineal massage religiously every evening for a half an hour. They are prepared because they are educated about the physical processes of pregnancy, labor, and birth; they are aware of the possibilities and have made their choices; they trust the mother's body, inner strength, and ability to give birth; they trust their relationship. Once prepared, they let things happen.

Childbirth is a unique event because it is one time in life when you are forced to be in the present. No planning tonight's dinner or thinking about your next career change. Contractions and the impending arrival force you to be in the now. That is as it should be, taking one contraction at a time and opening up to the new life inside. Linda did it consciously and at her own speed. So can you.

18

Anna

Postpartum Hemorrhage

At midnight, Anna was walking the halls. Her contractions were three minutes apart and a minute long. She was a tall, slender woman, graceful in her movements, not even noticeably pregnant when viewed from behind. She was walking fast, leaning on her husband, Carl, with each contraction. This was her second baby. Three-year-old Maggie was asleep at home with a baby-sitter.

Anna breathed heavily with each contraction, puffing and blowing in a pattern of her own design. She sighed at the end and smiled. She began walking again. After twenty minutes of this activity, she returned to her room to pee. As she stood up from the toilet, her waters broke, clear fluid running down her legs and puddling on the floor. A contraction started, and she leaned on me; Carl was in the other room.

"It's getting rough," she said.

"How about a shower?"

She stripped off her T-shirt and stepped under the hot spray. She leaned on the tile wall and puffed and blew with each contraction. Carl stood on the other side of the curtain, and I sat on the toilet. I listened to the baby's heartbeat periodically, getting soaked in the process. The water kept me awake at this late hour.

A few contractions later Anna said she had to push, and we headed for the bed. The doctor had arrived by now, and we stood by while Anna settled herself on the bed and began to push. She had marvelous gentle strength and a graceful presence, her long legs supported by slender hands. The mood in the room was joyful and wide awake even through it was nearing 1 A.M.

After three pushes, the head emerged and turned to ease the birth of the shoulders. Anna reached down for her second daughter, Elana. Elana opened her eyes and looked around. She began breathing without a sound— not a cry, not a whimper. She looked up at her parents, and Carl and Anna held her close.

"That was so much easier than last time!" said Anna. She went on to describe a thirty-six-hour labor with two hours of pushing. This time she had been in labor four hours, and Elana had been born after three brief pushes.

The cord stopped pulsing, was clamped and cut, and Elana began nursing. We waited patiently for the placenta. No sign of it yet—no little burst of blood or lengthening of the cord. No hurry, it had been less than ten minutes since the birth. The doctor examined Anna's perineum—just a superficial skin tear over the site of her episiotomy from Maggie's birth. No need for stitches.

I picked up instruments and wet blankets as we continued to wait for the placenta. Anna showed no signs of bleeding internally—her blood pressure and pulse were fine. I went to get her some juice.

When I returned, the doctor was tugging lightly on the cord. No movement. We waited some more. Elana switched to the other breast. It had been a half an hour since her birth. I was getting a little nervous about the lack of a placenta, and slipped out of the room to bring IV equipment just outside the door.

"Here it comes!" called the doctor as a gush of blood came from Anna's vagina, and the placenta followed close behind. The blood kept coming as the doctor laid his hand on her belly. Her uterus was not tightening, and the doctor asked me to give Anna a shot of Pitocin. Anna jumped as I inserted the needle into her thigh.

No help. The blood was still coming at a much faster pace than expected. Anna started to get pale. We moved into action. Suddenly the room was a flurry of activity as I lowered Anna so she lay flat in bed, another nurse handed Elana to Carl, and the doctor started an IV. I added Pitocin to the IV while the doctor returned to uterine massage. Carl sat in a chair with his daughter, looking frightened. Anna closed her eyes; her blood pressure had dropped from 120/72 to 90/50.

The IV was running in as fast as possible when the doctor put on fresh sterile gloves and put his hand into Anna's uterus. She barely moved as he swept her uterus for placental fragments and did bimanual compression, stopping the flow of blood by holding her uterus between his inside hand and his outside hand. The bleeding slowed. He removed his inner hand while keeping hold of her uterus with the hand on her belly. I gave her some Ergotrate, a stronger contracting drug than Pitocin. As this was going on, I attempted to calm Carl and explain what was happening.

Anna's bleeding had almost stopped, but she had lost several cups of blood. The doctor had found a small piece of placenta in her uterus, and with its removal the organ had been able to clamp down tightly to stop the flow of blood from the placental site. Her blood pressure had stabilized at 90/50 and her pulse at 110, I hung a second bottle of IV fluid. Elana slept peacefully in Carl's arms.

Anna lay still with her eyes closed, breathing peacefully. She would barely rouse when I spoke to her. The color slowly returned to her cheeks, and gradually her pulse lowered and her blood pressure rose. Carl handed Elana to me, and he went to Anna's side. He knelt by the side of the bed, held her hand, and whispered in her ear. I felt like an intruder on a very private scene, so I slipped into the chair in the corner, holding the peaceful, pink Elana.

"Will she be all right?" Carl asked.

"Yes," I said. "She's lost a lot of blood, but the bleeding has stopped now. She'll need to lie flat for a while and continue to have the IV. She may need a blood transfusion—we'll check for that later. She's going to need extra rest, iron, and fluids to replace what she's lost. But she'll be fine."

I knew she would be fine, but it had been a scary experience, as hemorrhages always are. They can happen so fast, and often with very little warning, as this one had.

After we settled Carl and Elana in for the night, the other nurse and I began to wash Anna. She was still sleeping peacefully with stable vital signs and minimal bleeding. But she was lying on wet, bloody sheets, and it was time to clean up. Carefully we rolled Anna from side to side, removing the dirty sheets, then washing her—back, legs, belly, crotch, blood was everywhere—and tucking in clean sheets under her. We got her T-shirt off and replaced it with a dry nightie. We washed her face and made her comfortable.

Thinking she was still asleep, we were shocked when Anna opened her eyes, smiled, and whispered, "Thank you."

*   *   *

Postpartum hemorrhage is a birth complication that is very frightening. Sometimes it can be predicted, but more often it cannot. It can happen slowly and insidiously or rapidly, as with Anna. It takes a fast-acting, well-prepared group of birth attendants to get a hemorrhage under control. Most home birth attendants carry IVs, Pitocin, and Ergotrate for just such rare circumstances. Things are a bit more comforting in a hospital—but just a bit.

Some women need surgery to remove all or part of a placenta that does not want to come out. Others may be helped by the bimanual compression done to Anna. IV fluids and drugs are a matter of course; blood transfusions less so since the discovery of the AIDS virus. But I have seen women with as many as three IVs—including blood—running into their arms, and surgeons and nurses working as fast as they can to stop the flow of lifeblood—whatever it takes to save a life.

Birth attendants and women can be prepared for the possibility of excessive bleeding if the labor is long and the uterus becomes tired; if the baby is very large (or there's more than one) and has stretched the uterus excessively, making it hard to contract; or if there is a family history of hemorrhage either with the woman's previous birth(s) or with her mother's births. Sometimes these women bleed too much and sometimes they don't—one more mystery in the dance of birth.

In any case, heavy bleeding needs to be slowed, and the woman can help by relaxing and letting the attendants do their work, visualizing her placenta coming out whole and her uterus stopping the flow of blood. Her partner can help by taking care of the baby—by holding, comforting, and warming the newborn. There is no need to separate the family even in this time of crisis. Unless the baby, too, is very ill, the mother's partner can provide a very important service by caring for the young child, who may be puzzled and startled by being removed from its mother. Again, the birth attendants need to reach a place of trust and action. Trust that the partner can care for the baby, trust that the woman will have the strength to live—and action in the form of all the medical procedures necessary to stop the bleeding.

In the case of a home birth, this situation may mean a hair-raising ride to the hospital in an ambulance. All the more reason for the attendants to be skilled and trusting and the partner to be a full participant. But with proper preparation—uterine-contracting drugs, fluid replacement in the form of IVs or enemas, skills in bimanual compression, posted phone numbers of the ambulance and hospital—a hemorrhage can be handled safely. Hemorrhages are rare but, like other complications, can happen. Careful, competent birth attendants—at home or in the hospital—need to be ready for any possible danger.

Should you, as a pregnant woman, be afraid of postpartum hemorrhage? No; it is rare. Better to put your energies toward good health, keeping up the iron level in your blood—that will help whether or not you hemorrhage—and finding a well-trained birth attendant. Put your trust in your body, in your power and your strength, knowing that even if you do bleed excessively, your body will be able to heal itself.

19

Penny

Holding Back

The phone rang at 9 A.M. I was at home, just finishing the breakfast dishes, and answered the phone with wet hands. It was Penny. She was due sometime this month with her second child. She had never had a period between weaning her first child and getting pregnant again. By her estimation she was due now; by measurement, movement, and first-heard heartbeat, the doctor placed her two weeks later. In any case, her waters had just broken.

I had attended Penny's first birth, her daughter Tina—a planned home birth that ended up in the hospital for meconium-stained fluid. All had gone well, and Tina and her parents had gone home two hours after her birth.

Now, two years later, Penny and Dan had planned this birth at home. It was a lovely day in July. Penny wasn't having any contractions yet, and I told her not to worry about it, things would start soon enough. We planned to keep in touch.

Two hours later I called. No contractions. Dan said they were busy getting things ready—doing some baking, playing with Tina, cleaning the house, and waiting for his mother to arrive. Dan and Penny had decided that they did not want Tina at the birth and had enlisted the help of Dan's mother to care for her during the labor and birth. However, she was six hours and two states away. I suggested they might want to have a backup child care person, but they said no, they'd wait for Grandma.

I tried to keep busy and not get anxious about the impending birth. I wanted to get going, to be there, but I knew there was no reason for my presence. I worked in my garden, played with my daughter, and spoke with the doctor. She was concerned about the lack of labor and suggested we push Penny and Dan to try some breast stimulation.

Phone calls at 2 P.M. and 4 P.M. yielded the same answer—no labor and very little fluid. Maybe it wasn't really time after all. The doctor and I agreed to meet them to do a sterile speculum exam to check the fluid—maybe it wasn't amniotic fluid but a heavy vaginal discharge instead.

Everyone arrived at once: Grandma drove up right behind the doctor, and I came a minute later. There were a few hectic moments, then Grandma took Tina for a walk while we did the exam. Yes, it was amniotic fluid, and Penny looked to be about three centimeters dilated. I decided to stay, and the doctor went home to give her kids supper.

Grandma unpacked and Tina was hopping around the house, unwrapping presents. Dan and Penny tried to get supper. There was a definite feeling of confusion in the house, and Tina was doing a great job of acting it out—she would hardly sit still for a minute. After everyone had eaten, Dan and Penny decided to take Tina for a walk, hoping to tire her out and stimulate labor at the same time. Grandma and I settled down to read.

An hour later they returned. No contractions, but it was time for bed. The family went through their bedtime rituals while I tried to stay out of the way. Pajamas, stories, kisses, and Tina was tucked into bed. We all breathed a sigh of relief. It was nine o'clock.

Dan and Penny went upstairs to work on stimulating labor—some passionate kissing and breast stimulation usually got things going. I went back to reading. Ten minutes later I heard noises from upstairs—the unmistakable sounds of a woman in labor. At the same time Tina opened her door and peeked out. She was not interested in going to sleep. Grandma and I tried to play with her, but she wanted Mama. Dan and Penny heard the commotion and came downstairs.

They tried reading her another book. It was difficult for Penny, who was having contractions, to hold Tina on her lap as Dan read the story. Penny did her best to get through each contraction without disturbing Tina, but after a couple of contractions Penny stood up and began walking around.

Dan took Tina back to her bed and tried lying down with her. Penny's contractions picked up speed, and she began moaning with each one. Dan and Tina emerged from the bedroom and went outside. The noise was too distracting for her, so Grandma took her for another walk, this time in starlight.

For the next hour Dan went back and forth between Penny and Tina, trying to calm his sobbing daughter and support his laboring wife. I stayed with Penny, and in time called the doctor to tell her things were happening. Penny stayed on her hands and knees, leaning on a great pile of pillows, moaning with each contraction. The volume of the moans increased in direct proportion to the intensity of the contractions.

Between contractions Penny would ask me about Tina. Could I hear her? Was she still crying? What were they doing out there?

For a short time Penny had no contractions as she fretted

about Tina. I finally said, "You've got to stop thinking about Tina. You've got a new child who needs you now, who needs you to pay attention to your labor. This child wants to get born. Tina will be OK with her grandmother, she's being taken care of. Let's get this baby born."

The contractions resumed, and Penny had a determined look on her face. The contractions were long and strong, and Penny cried out at the peak. She finally insisted that Dan stay with her. Grandma held Tina in the front seat of her car—the house was too small to find a quiet place for Tina—and gradually her sobs slowed and she was quiet. About that time the doctor arrived, and Penny said she felt pressure.

The only sound now was the low sigh of Penny's pushing. She turned over with the pillow pile at her back, knees held by arms, and gently pushed. The doctor and Dan were on the floor at the edge of the bed, and I was up with Penny, supporting the pillows as much as Penny. Gradually we began to see wisps of hair, then a wrinkled scalp, and the head was born. Together, Dan and the doctor held the baby as he was born and laid him on Penny's belly. It was 11 P.M.

I dried Ted off and covered him and Penny with warm blankets. Dan crawled up on the bed with them. A gush of blood heralded the arrival of the placenta, which was born after a small push. However, the blood kept coming and Penny's uterus was not contracting. I gave her a shot of Pitocin while the doctor massaged her belly, and Penny tried to put Ted to breast. Within a few minutes her bleeding slowed and Ted began to nurse. We cleaned up.

Dan went out to the car, told his mother of the birth, and carried a now soundly sleeping Tina to bed. Grandma came in and admired her new grandson. After one last check of Penny's still-firm uterus, the other midwife and I went into the other room to give the family some time together.

An hour later I was on my way home, happy that Tina

had a brother and that Dan and Penny had had this baby at home.

* * *

What had happened in Penny's body that day? Was it simply that her labor would not begin without stimulation, or was it something else? Was she holding back, waiting? Waiting for the right time—the arrival of Grandma, Tina's bedtime, a time when she could be relaxed and ready to labor?

Later, I talked with Penny about Ted's birth. I brought up my idea that she had controlled when her labor would start. Penny understood perfectly.

"Oh, sure," she said. "I knew I didn't want to have that baby 'til Grandma was there and Tina was asleep. I needed to have that to be able to relax and try the stimulation and go into labor. I knew exactly what I was doing."

I was amazed and pleased to hear Penny being so clear about what had happened. Time and again I had seen women in labor who were clearly controlling what was happening. Some had held back, others had forged ahead when complications threatened. One woman had dilated seven centimeters in ten minutes as we were setting up for a cesarean. I knew it could be done, and I was thrilled to speak to a woman who was aware of her control.

The women who got stuck at a certain place in their labor—most commonly somewhere between six and eight centimeters—needed to have the right circumstances to move on. Sometimes those circumstances were a change in mind-set or a change in physical surroundings. Perhaps they needed to be somewhere else to get "unstuck," sometimes they needed to have more or fewer people with them, some needed to be alone with their partner, others didn't want their partner near. Some women would be open to talking about what was holding them back, others wanted no words.

Although this emotional/physical link is well known to

midwives, few doctors subscribe to it. Most doctors insist that a cesarean done for "failure to progress" is based solely on a physical problem—a baby that is too big or in the wrong position. But I expect they are wrong. "Failure to progress" is the same as "unable to open up." A woman may be unable to open up to her fear of pain, to the reality of having to drip bodily fluids in front of strangers, to becoming a mother, to continuing a failing relationship with her partner. She may have unconscious fears of being ripped open, of losing control, of making sexual-sounding noises.

To give birth you must lose control, give in, allow it to happen. You must accept your noises, your body, your fluids, your words. This society does not provide many opportunities to lose control, to be truly in your body, and to be completely in the present. Making love and having orgasms is one way. Some people have compared it to taking a drug such as LSD. You have to "go with it" to achieve orgasm. You have to "go with it" or you'll have a "bad trip." You have to "go with it" to give birth.

Birth attendants can do many things to help a woman "go with it"—from talking about it to asking her partner to leave the room. But ultimately the woman has to take responsibility for her own behavior, she has to reach down inside of herself and "give in." Penny needed to give up her need to take care of Tina in order to take care of herself and the baby who was trying to be born. Other women have to give up their particular needs and fears to focus on the present, the labor, the birth.

Yes, there are some physical reasons for cesareans, forceps, episiotomies, IVs, certain medications. But I expect that these interventions are used more often for psychological needs—those of the birth attendant or the laboring woman. The time for women to deal with their issues is during (or before) pregnancy. But often they are not aware of them until labor begins. A sensitive birth attendant who becomes aware during prenatal care of possible blocks can deal with them then. The time for birth attendants to deal with their own issues—malpractice suits, impatience, fear of deviating from routine, discomfort with women expressing pain and making sexual noises—is *now,* before they push any more of their fears onto the laboring woman.

All laboring women deserve to give birth at their own speed, in their own way. Birth attendants are there to ensure safe passage and to encourage women to open up to their place of power and strength, to give up that which they cannot change, and allow their babies to make the passage into this world. Birth attendants do not deliver babies but should be there to help the women do what they know how to do—give birth.

20

Sally

A Woman-Chosen Pitocin Induction

Sally's two girls were five and eight. They had both been born at a large medical center after an induced labor when Sally was past forty-two weeks. Sally's labors had never started on their own—some mystery in her body had prevented spontaneous labor. Or was it the doctors who said the babies must be born at forty-two weeks, no more, because of possible complications? (There's a greater chance of the placenta deciding to quit work by then, with problems resulting because of lack of oxygen for the baby, mainly fetal distress and meconium staining of the fluid.) On top of her inductions, Sally had endured "high-tech" births associated with Pitocin inductions at some institutions—continuous fetal monitoring and delivery room deliveries. Sally's two girls had been healthy, but she had been disappointed and longed for a natural birth.

When Sally became pregnant again, she and her husband, Jack, had been thrilled. Since she was a friend of mine, she appeared one day in early pregnancy and asked me if I could hear the baby's heartbeat. I searched her belly with the Doptone and found one, just above the pubic hair line. After this exciting beginning, I spent time with her throughout her pregnancy, and she spoke with me of her desire for the birth.

She wanted the baby to be born before forty-two weeks so there would not be the added stress of worrying about its condition. So at forty weeks she began her private induction campaign. Her doctor had approved but had warned her that nothing might come of it. First she and Jack tried lots and lots of sex, but there were no signs of labor. Then she moved on to castor oil, which did nothing but give her diarrhea. She was ready for Pitocin, and her doctor agreed.

At forty-one weeks she came to the birthing center one day while I was working. I started the IV and increased the dosage of Pitocin every fifteen minutes, waiting for contractions. When I had reached the maximum dosage and held it there for a couple of hours, we finally decided to turn it off. Not a twinge. Sally's uterus did not budge—this baby was not ready to come out.

A few more days went by, and Sally's anxiety increased measurably. She finally decided to try the Pitocin again, this time having her waters broken at the same time. She was sure that would guarantee labor. She was already four centimeters dilated, so breaking the waters would be easy. She picked her night, and we all assembled at the birthing center.

Sally and Jack had enjoyed a gourmet dinner at the home of friends and arrived at the center around 9 P.M. I was to attend this birth as a friend along with Helena, another friend of Sally and Jack's. The doctor, the nurse on duty, and Sally and Jack's older girls completed the scene.

By 9:30 the IV had been started and, as before, the Pitocin did not seem to be doing anything. At 10:15 Sally asked the doctor to break her waters, and he did; the fluid was clear. The mood in the room was light. I sat on the bed with Helena and Sally, talking. The girls were cuddling in their father's lap. Then, *wham!* About five minutes after the waters were broken, Sally's labor began.

What happened next was a roller-coaster ride of a labor.

The contractions came fast and furious, and Sally did her best to go with them. The Pitocin dosage was never increased again, and actually was very low. Helena and Jack and I stayed with Sally, spoke with her, and supplied her with ice water, cold washcloths, and words of encouragement. The contractions had come on so rapidly and so intensely that she could not move from her sitting position on the double bed. At a few minutes before eleven she said, "Here comes the baby!" and she pushed.

With one fast push the baby slithered out onto the bed, wet and squalling. Another girl! The doctor lifted her out of the puddle and handed her to Sally. Rowan's screams were as loud as the laughter in the room. Her sisters climbed up on the bed to see her. After Sally's placenta came and her bleeding had slowed, we turned off the Pitocin and took out the IV. Sally was radiant, surrounded by her family; Rowan was eagerly, almost voraciously, nursing.

Somebody popped a bottle of champagne, and we stayed until midnight, celebrating. Then Jack took the girls home, and Helena and I disappeared into the night.

In the morning when I arrived at work, Sally was up with Rowan, as she had been half the night. Rowan loved to nurse so much that Sally was sore and tired. But she was happy. She was so pleased that she had had such a pleasant labor. She was glad to have been surrounded by friends and to have had her baby in bed—no stitches, no problems.

"It was such a great feeling in the room," she said. "I mean, that labor was pretty fast and pretty intense, but knowing that all of you were with me made it worth it. What a great way to have a baby!"

*   *   *

Pitocin induction. A nasty phrase in some circles and a possibly dangerous procedure as well. But in Sally's case (and Laura's in Chapter 7) Pitocin was the answer to her particular needs, in this case getting the baby born before forty-two weeks. Some might think that would be negatively manipulating Rowan's appearance or that Sally had a psychological block to going into labor on her own. Perhaps. The important thing here is that Sally *chose* the Pitocin; it was not forced on her, as it had been the two previous times. This was a woman-centered and woman-controlled labor and birth. Sally did what she did to get her needs met.

She often joked later about Rowan getting "ejected," and that was true. Rowan did not come in her own time— or did she? Sally's previous induction attempts had not worked. This time they did. Since no one completely understands the link between the baby and the beginning of labor, you could argue that it was fine with Rowan. In any case, Sally was sure of her time of conception and when we had first heard the heartbeat, so there was no fear of Rowan's being too early. That can be one of the greatest dangers of induction.

Often inductions are done at the convenience of the doctor—Monday morning, for instance. Most hospitals have the policy that a doctor needs to be on the hospital premises when Pitocin is running, so he or she may find it convenient to order an induction in the daytime if his or her office is on the hospital grounds. Doctors who have to come in for an induction often run out of patience and turn the drug up too fast, too soon, to "get things going," or stop the process too soon if it is not going quickly enough for them.

Pitocin, used at the right time, with the right attitude, can be a useful drug to help a labor that has stopped or slowed if there is no time or interest in using other methods to stimulate labor. It can also be useful to start a labor that is not starting on its own—for whatever reason—if the request comes from the woman and she is on or past her due date.

Pitocin does not have to go hand in hand with other birth technology—mainly continuous fetal monitoring. Most hospitals have the policy that if Pitocin is running, the fetal monitor has to be running as well. This shows how dangerous Pitocin is considered to be. It can produce prolonged, strong contractions that can be too much for a baby to handle, thus causing severe fetal distress. But a well-trained, sensitive nurse can monitor the baby and the quality of contractions with her ear and her hand as well as, if not better than, the monitor. This allows the woman to get up and move around, walk, take a shower, use the toilet—whatever will make her more comfortable. If the goal is to get a labor going well, then its makes sense to do all those other things to help the woman. Being forced to stay in bed with an IV and two monitor belts attached to a pregnant belly can increase not only the pain but also the woman's anxiety level. A greater anxiety level may increase the likelihood of not opening up, as well as the possibility of fetal distress.

By all means use Pitocin, if that seems to be the only answer. But use it carefully, cautiously, and with respect. An IV need not restrain a woman from doing anything she might otherwise do in her labor. It is a portable tool. A nurse's continuous presence should not hinder a woman either, if the nurse is respectful and watchful, either staying discreetly out of the way or stepping in to help the woman, if that is what she needs. The point here is respect—respect for the drug's power, respect for the woman's power, respect for the power of birth. The birth attendants should hold that foremost as they consider, with the woman and her partner, the use of Pitocin. It need not detract from a woman-centered, joyous birth. It can be a useful appropriate technology when used at the right time and in the right way.

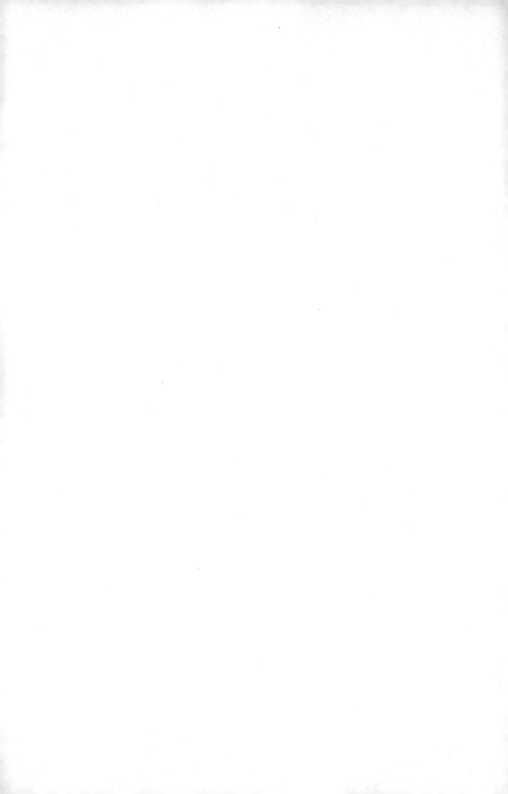

21

Lynn

Gestational Diabetic

At the birthing center we knew Lynn well. She had given birth to five children and was now pregnant with her sixth. During this pregnancy she had been in and out of the center several times. She had been diagnosed a gestational diabetic, unable to handle sugar in her system without the help of daily injections of insulin. She stayed with us to learn how to test her blood sugar, give herself insulin shots, and eat a balanced diet. Lynn was a happy, warm woman, and we loved having her around. Her husband, Roger, visited her religiously every evening, and we would see them cuddling on her bed. It was nice to know romance could still be alive after so many children!

Lynn's previous babies had gotten bigger and bigger in size; her last one had weighed over thirteen pounds and had some blood sugar problems after birth. Lynn's midwife watched her carefully throughout this pregnancy and shared Lynn's care with a doctor when the diabetes was diagnosed. We hoped this baby would not be so big or so sick.

Lynn, Roger, the doctor, and the midwife conferred often. They decided to induce labor at about thirty-eight weeks to make sure the baby and the placenta were strong enough to handle the contractions. Often a diabetic's placenta is not as efficient an organ for providing oxygen and filtering waste from the baby as the placenta of a nondiabetic woman.

Lynn and Roger picked an evening when his parents could stay with the other children and planned to start the induction about 8 P.M. The doctor hoped to induce simply by breaking Lynn's waters and thereby avoid Pitocin; Lynn was three centimeters dilated. The doctor also insisted that Lynn have continuous monitoring with an electronic fetal monitor.

Everyone assembled a little before eight. The doctor successfully broke Lynn's waters and screwed the internal monitor lead into the baby's head. The thump-thump-thump sounded clearly in the room, and the printout rolled with a squiggly line that indicated the variations in the heartbeat. Lynn got up, sat in a rocking chair, and rocked.

Fifteen minutes went by, and she began to have a few mild contractions. I got a long extension cord for the monitor, and while Lynn and Roger walked up and down the hall, I pushed the machine, tended the cords, and mopped the floor where she dripped clear fluid. The contractions began to get stronger, and she returned to her room.

All of a sudden the contractions were two minutes apart and a minute long. Roger, the midwife, and I crowded into the bathroom, where Lynn sat rocking on the toilet. She held her belly and swayed silently with each contraction. The doctor sat in the other room, waiting. We stayed with Lynn, rubbed her back, and wiped her brow with cool washcloths.

At a few minutes to nine, Lynn said she felt pressure, and we helped her back to the bed. Before the midwife could check her, she started to push. We watched the internal monitor lead come out of her vagina, knowing the baby's head was close behind. The baby's heartbeat was still strong, and the midwife unscrewed the lead as the head emerged, dark and wet. The baby slithered out into her hands, and she lifted Abby onto Lynn's belly while Roger held his wife. Abby squalled and pinked up. I dried her and covered her with warm blankets. She looked to be about seven pounds, healthy and vigorous.

Roger and Lynn now had three girls and three boys, and were delighted with their new addition. Lynn, an old hand at nursing, put Abby to her breast. The placenta came easily, already showing signs of calcification—roughened areas that had stopped working. Lynn's perineum showed no signs of the recent birth, and her bleeding was minimal.

After another day in the hospital to check both Lynn's and Abby's blood sugar levels, they went home to join the rest of the family. We would miss Lynn and her cheerful presence, but we were glad that everything had gone well for her and Abby. Lynn's blood sugar problems had ended as abruptly as her pregnancy.

*   *   *

This short and simple story of Abby's birth tells little of all the vials of blood, the seemingly endless monitor paper from Lynn's daily non-stress tests, and the nights Lynn stayed in the hospital away from her family. Today's technology has helped the pre-pregnant diabetic as well as the pregnancy-induced diabetic to have a healthy pregnancy and a healthy baby. However, having such a condition does not necessarily mean a high-tech birth.

Lynn and Roger knew that the doctor felt it was best to induce labor early. But the doctor did not make the final decision; it was left to Lynn and Roger to pick when and where. The doctor agreed to play a secondary role at the birth, leaving labor support and baby "catching" to the midwife. Except for the relentless bleeps and thumps emanating from the fetal monitor, Lynn's labor and birth were hardly different from the others I attended every day.

Lynn did not stay in her room; she walked when she wanted and sat when she wanted. She had support from her husband, her midwife, and her nurse. She gave birth in the bed with no episiotomy, no rushing the baby away "to make sure she was all right." We could observe Abby with our eyes—watch her vigor, her color, her alertness—and be vigilant and ready to step in if necessary. Other than the wires that came from her vagina, attached to her thigh, and hooked to the machine, Lynn looked like any other woman in labor.

Technology is vitally important in some cases. We were well prepared with IVs, resuscitation equipment, various medicines, blood testing supplies—everything to assure Lynn's and Abby's good health and safety. But nothing was used without a good reason. I did not fully agree with the doctor's desire to use the fetal monitor—I still feel a baby can be properly monitored by a competent birth attendant with a fetoscope or Doptone—but since it was going to be used, I did what I could to make it comfortable and unobtrusive for Lynn.

Perhaps that is another lesson for birth attendants—if technology is to be used, it should be made as comfortable and unobtrusive for the woman as possible. IVs can be very portable; I've had plenty in the shower. Fetal monitors can be adjusted to allow a woman to walk or sit during her labor. Emergency supplies can be set up within reach but out of sight. And anything that is done or used should be discussed with the woman and her partner first.

Even in the rush to correct a severe complication, things can be explained to the parents. There should be enough birth attendants available to allow one to remain at the mother's side and explain the situation. More than once I have stood next to a woman as I helped push the gurney to the operating room and said, "The baby's heartbeat is very low" or "You're losing a lot of blood, we need to stop it," in as reassuring a voice as possible. Phrases like "I'll stay with you and be right here when you wake up" or "I'll be taking care of your baby when it is born" can be comforting to a woman who may be terrified of the rapid change in circumstances and fear the unknown.

Complication: what does it mean? Some pregnancies and births have life-threatening problems; others have incidents out of the ordinary as defined by the medical model of birth—"too long" or "too short" labors or pushing times, labors that slow or stop and need to be prodded into resuming, a baby in a posterior position (facing the mother's belly instead of her back), and waters that are broken for more than twenty-four hours, for example.

In the midwifery model there is no sense of "ordinary" and "not ordinary," only a continuum on which a woman and her baby may fall anywhere. The midwife encourages the woman to listen to her body and her inner power, and to birth her baby the way she knows best. The midwife is aware of possible life-threatening situations and is always ready to ensure a safe passage. But she mostly sits back, observes, and gives the woman the space and encouragement to find her own strength.

Even in complicated situations the midwifery model can take precedence, continually respecting the laboring woman's place at the center of the mystery of birth. Women like Lynn can have their medical problems cared for yet maintain their self-esteem and control over the birth of their child. Birth attendants need to learn to combine their technical expertise with empathic and respectful care so that all women can give birth as they know best.

22

Tammy

Stuck at Eight

Tammy had struggled with the decision to have a second child. At times, she felt smothered by motherhood and longed to have some time to herself. She spoke with me often about her dilemma and eventually decided to become pregnant. Her daughter Emma was three.

I remember when Emma was born. Tammy and her partner, Barry, had wanted a home birth. It was a snowy day in January when we assembled for Emma's birth. Tammy had started labor around four in the morning, and her waters had broken soon after that. After three hours of labor, she was five centimeters dilated; after another three hours, she was eight to nine, but the head was still high.

She seemed to be enjoying labor and excited that her first child was soon to be born. She walked around stark naked except for a wet washcloth draped over her head. When she had a contraction, she leaned on Barry or one of the midwives. After another hour she started making pushing sounds and sat on the birthing chair to push. She said it didn't feel right, and one of the midwives checked her. She was now seven centimeters, but the head was lower. Tammy was very disappointed. She had been in labor nine hours and had expected her baby soon.

For the next few hours Tammy and Barry and the midwives did everything to help Tammy open up—she showered, she danced, she squatted, she walked, she was
catheterized for being unable to pee. As the afternoon
wore on, she was still seven centimeters, maybe eight, but
the cervix was swelling with the pressure of the head,
which was much lower. At 5 P.M. the midwives heard
some slowing of the baby's heartbeat, and the decision
was made to go to the hospital.

Into the snowstorm they went, Barry driving and
Tammy on all fours in the back of the station wagon. The
midwives had oxygen and the birth kit in case things
changed. Because of the snow, the hospital was forty-five
minutes away. Tammy struggled with each contraction,
wanting desperately to push each time because of the
pressure. The midwives coached her through each contraction, breathing with her to keep her from pushing. The
baby's heartbeat rebelled with each push by dropping but
recovered well when the pressure stopped.

At the hospital the doctor checked Tammy. Now she was
a good eight centimeters, and the cervix had softened
some and had lost its swelling. Between contractions, they
talked about what to do. Then the heartbeat began to slow
even more. Tammy lay in bed on her left side, an IV was
started, and she breathed oxygen through a cup. The surgical team was notified for a possible cesarean, but it
would take them at least a half an hour to be ready.

Then the doctor made a radical suggestion.

"You know, Tammy, the baby's head is so low I can practically see it when I spread your labia. Why don't you try
pushing with the contraction and I'll work on stretching
your cervix?"

So the pattern began—Tammy would push, the doctor
would spread her cervix with his fingers. It seemed to be
working. But the baby did not like it—the heartbeat would
drop to eighty with each push and would slowly recover

as Tammy breathed the oxygen. The pattern changed to push with one contraction and breathe through the next. The baby liked this new pattern much better.

After doing this for twenty minutes or so, the doctor said, "The cervix is gone, go ahead and push." Tammy took a deep breath and pushed. The midwives were encouraging her, and Barry was holding her.

"That's good, I can see the head. Keep it coming. Wait, wait, slow down, slow down, stop pushing! Let me suction the baby!"

"No, I'm not stopping now," said Tammy, and in one push Emma was born. Tammy reached down for her and held her at her breast. Tammy, Barry, and Emma were all crying, and the rest of us in the room were very relieved. Emma was fine and, so it seemed, was Tammy. Soon the placenta came, and the doctor checked Tammy's perineum—hardly a scratch.

Now that Tammy was pregnant again, she was sure the same thing would not happen a second time. She knew that second babies come faster than first babies and actually, as stressful as Emma's labor had been, it had only been a little under fourteen hours, quite "average" for a first baby. She and Barry planned another home birth, found some midwives to help, and a friend, Charlotte, to care for Emma. I was to attend as a friend.

Emma was well prepared throughout the pregnancy and picked her role for the birth. It was to be her job to check the baby's gender and to get the baby's blankets. Tammy did not enjoy being pregnant as much as she had the first time, but she grew to love the quiet little child that floated in her womb.

At 7 A.M. on a warm fall day she called me. The contractions had started at 6 A.M. and were five minutes apart. The midwives were on their way.

By the time everyone had assembled, Tammy was in the bathroom, leaning on a counter and breathing a low, chanting moan with each contraction. She clutched a pile of cold, wet washcloths. Emma played quietly in the other room with Charlotte and checked in on her mother every once in a while.

At 9 A.M. Tammy was five centimeters dilated, at 11 A.M. she was seven, at 1 P.M. she was eight to nine but the head was still high. We discussed the pros and cons of breaking her waters. Tammy wanted things to hurry up and thought that the head would come down and her cervix would open right up with the pressure. She pushed for breaking. The midwives were reluctant because the head was so high, but Tammy insisted, so everyone piled onto the bed. The amnihook's sharp point burst the bubble, the fluid gushed out, and the head came down. But now Tammy was six centimeters. She was devastated.

Tammy cried and sobbed and hollered "Why me?" and "This isn't fair! Second babies are supposed to be faster!" We did what we could to console her in between the contractions that were coming faster. Tammy insisted that the midwife try to push her cervix open, and after a few attempts, the midwife stopped, saying the cervix was tight, and was only getting swollen. Tammy held Barry and cried for a while. The rest of us sat silent, and Charlotte took Emma outside to play.

Then one of the midwives spoke up. "You just need more time, Tammy, your cervix isn't ready. You just have to accept that you need to open more—and *you* need to do the work. Let's go outside."

Into the sunny day they went. There was a light breeze, and everyone but Tammy needed a sweater. Tammy was naked, sitting on a chair under a tree. She became quiet—no chatting between contractions—but moaned louder with each contraction. She buried her head in Barry's waist while he held her.

"I don't want to do this anymore. I can't stand this, it hurts. What's wrong with me?" Tammy began to wail. The midwife spoke calmly to her, telling her to let go, let it happen, to visualize her cervix opening. Tammy buried her head in Barry's waist again, her arms around him, and was silent.

For another hour they sat there, quiet in the fall breeze. The only sound was Tammy's deep moans with each contraction. Then Tammy asked to be checked.

"You're eight now," said the midwife. "And the head is much lower."

"Can I push now?" asked Tammy. "Try pushing my cervix open like last time."

They tried a few contractions out there in the yard, Tammy pushing and the midwife stretching her cervix inside. It started to work. The cervix was soft, and it was opening. We all went back to the bed.

Tammy seemed happier to push. Even though she said it hurt, she said it didn't hurt as much as "just sitting around" with the contractions. This baby was handling the pushing well—no drop in the heartbeat.

After a dozen contractions Tammy cried, "It's about to go, I can feel it, the cervix is going!" Charlotte and Emma scurried into the room. Barry knelt between Tammy's legs and, with some guidance from the midwife, held the baby's head as it emerged in one big push. Tammy pushed again, and the shoulders and body slithered out into Barry's hands. Tammy reached down to take the baby from Barry, and Emma scrambled up onto the bed with the blankets.

She covered the baby and then peeked under the blankets. "It's a boy!" she announced. Everyone laughed, and Barry joined Emma at Tammy's side. Galen was spluttering and blinking, trying to open his eyes in the sunny room. His gray-purple color rapidly changed to pink as he breathed in his new surroundings. Once again the placenta came easily, and Tammy's perineum was intact. We celebrated with champagne and supper, and after a couple of hours left the family happily snuggling on the bed, calling friends and relatives.

*   *   *

Tammy's worst nightmare had come true—her second labor was almost the same as her first. With the exception of the home-to-hospital transfer and Emma's low heartbeat, the same scenario repeated itself. Why? Was there some physical abnormality in Tammy's cervix, some odd pelvic structure that kept the baby's head high? Or was she simply holding back, afraid of the pain, afraid of the opening, unable or unwilling to do it without help?

We'll never know about the physical structure of Tammy's cervix and pelvis. I had seen cervixes shrink before, but never to this extreme. I knew it was common for women to have blocks that held their cervix in one place for a long time and that they needed to break through their block or risk a surgical birth. Sometimes their blocks were caused by fear of pain, fear of motherhood, a failing relationship with their partner. But I knew that Tammy was thrilled to be having Emma, had dreamed a long time about motherhood, and that once she made her decision to become pregnant again, had the same excitement. She and Barry were deeply in love. She wasn't crazy about the pain but had handled it well in both labors—until the point where she became stuck.

Tammy and I had many conversations about her labors. It disturbed her that she couldn't open on her own. But knowing her as well as I did, I offered another theory. Tammy was a woman who liked to be in control of things in her life. As long as her labors were going her way, she was happy, she was in control. But once they wavered from her script, she became angry, frustrated—and stuck. She also had a hard time letting people take care of her. As her friend, I watched her care for others—friends, relatives, animals—but she had a hard time asking for help for herself.

Tammy needed a combination of being in control and being helped to open up and give birth. Both times those needs manifested themselves in the combination of her pushing and her birth attendant opening her cervix manually—she was in control *and* she was being helped. The process worked. Who knows what might have happened with different birth attendants, who might have insisted she do it herself or have offered pain medication or have packed her off to surgery? But, as with so many other circumstances, wondering "what if?" doesn't tell us any more than considering the facts.

I'm sure that those birth attendants who follow the medical model of birth would be appalled by my psychological interpretation of Emma's and Galen's births. They would boil it all down to a cervix that just did not want to work—and would be sure that an epidural and some Pitocin would have been the answer to the problem. They would say that the contractions weren't working properly and that a little Pitocin would straighten them out—as long as Tammy had an epidural so she would be relaxed enough to let the Pitocin do its work.

What would have been the harm in such an alternative? It would no longer be Tammy's body giving birth, but the medicine and the doctor doing the work. Her babies would have been born, yes, but where would the satisfaction be? Tammy was already disturbed by her labors; she might have become even more upset if they had been taken away from her altogether. I often wonder if some forms of postpartum depression are caused by feelings of labor and birth loss—loss of awareness, loss of plans, loss of control, loss of contact with the body, loss of contact with the baby. Besides, once Tammy talked through her concerns about her labors with both me and Barry, she began to see her control and caring-for needs more clearly and finally gained resolution, as well as increased self-awareness.

Perhaps other women are not as ready or able to work

on their inner selves as Tammy was. Perhaps they would be happier with epidurals and doctor-orchestrated births. But I know Tammy, as well as many other women, who feel powerful in their bodies, who know their strength as women and use it. I also have been with countless women who started their labors without an inkling of their power and emerged with a new vision of themselves, a vision of a strong woman who is capable of doing one of the most challenging things in the world—giving birth. It gave them a taste of possibilities, and I would not have wanted to deny them that experience.

As birth attendants we must be careful of blaming women when they are unable to tap into that inner power. If women get stuck and do not open, even with all our visualizations and psychological theorizing, then we need to support them through surgery or whatever interventions are necessary. Sometimes intervening is the only way to get the baby born. But if we sense they are ready or open to talking about psychological and emotional factors in their labors, then by all means we should go ahead. Our choices must be based on our respect for the laboring woman and her personal strengths and weaknesses.

As laboring women we must be open to emotional blockage factors as well as physical complications and to our choices for solving those problems. When we educate ourselves about pregnancy, labor, and birth, we must look at all aspects. It is a marvelous time to open up to the inner self and listen. Learning more about how you tick, your triggers, and your issues can only make you a more whole person in the end, more able to care for your self, more able to be a loving, trusting partner, more able to be a patient parent. After all, the labor and birth of a child are only a minute part of parenthood. There are so many more challenges to come!

Tammy was able to learn more about herself and her needs. She was happy to have been surrounded by friends and birth attendants who cared enough to help her work it out. Perhaps you can do the same for yourself or other laboring women. At times, we all are laboring with something attempting to emerge—not necessarily a baby trying to come out of a womb. Birth time is no different from other times in our life when we may need a midwife to help us in our labors. We can all learn to be midwives for each other—and for our selves—so we can become "unstuck" and grow.

23

Women-Centered Birth

To the Pregnant Woman

You have embarked upon one of the most challenging journeys of life: parenthood. You have also embarked upon another great journey of life: choosing to give space within you to the child you will parent, and then to give birth to that child. The nine months of pregnancy and the brief hours of labor are only a speck of time compared with a lifetime of parenting. It is a thought to remember.

The months of pregnancy are extraordinarily important. They give you the time to prepare to become a parent, to care for yourself as a way of caring for the child within your womb, to educate yourself about your body, the child's body, and the beginnings of life. The months also give you the time to choose—to choose your birth attendants and place of birth, to choose the way you want to help your child move from womb to arms. Remember, not only will you be birthing a baby, you will be giving birth to yourself as a parent.

Women have been embarking upon this rite of passage since the beginning of time. Women nurture life within and open up to allow the child a place in the world. Women have always surrounded other women during pregnancy, birth, and the early months of babyhood and parenthood. This passage is important enough to make a conscious decision about those women who will surround you.

If you are fortunate enough to live in an area where you have a long list of choices, be sure to examine them carefully. Decide if home or hospital is best for you. If you choose home, be sure to find a compatible midwife and work closely with her to ensure a safe and healthy birth.

If you choose a hospital, decide if you want a small community hospital, a birthing center, or a high-tech institution. Where will you be most comfortable? Go to each institution and look around, ask questions of staff members. Get a feel for the place. If you are refused a tour or find the staff members busy telling you what will happen to you without a sense of flexibility, you would be wise to look elsewhere. Since the nurses are the people you will be spending the most time with, see if you like them—talk with the head nurse or nurse manager and find out the prevailing attitude. Beautiful furniture and flowered wallpaper are not enough—you're looking for respect and care for you, your partner, and your child. That comes not with the surroundings but with the people.

It is a time to look within and be honest with yourself. How do you feel about pain? Do you know how to relax? Do you trust your body? Do you trust your partner? Now is the time for therapy, exercise, meditation, or other types of self-help if you feel you need it. Pregnancy is a time of growth not just for the baby but for the future parents as well. The person you choose to provide your prenatal care can assist you to find the help you need.

Don't be afraid to change. If you don't like your chosen birth attendant, find a new one, even if it is your eighth or ninth month. Try to do it sooner, and you'll save everyone—especially yourself—a lot of stress. Your comfort level is paramount, and if you aren't being treated the way you would like, find someone else. If you have no choices in your area, talk it out with your birth attendant and make a list of your wants and needs. Remember, your birth attendant is working for *you*—you pay the bills, you do the hiring and the firing, you hold the power.

Educate yourself, but don't go overboard—you're not cramming for the obstetrical boards. Read, ask questions, talk with your friends, go to childbirth classes. But don't let anyone tell you that if you breathe a certain way, there will be no pain. Childbirth classes are for learning to relax and open up to the strength inside, not for puffing and blowing in certain patterns.

Make a birth plan. List the things you want and don't want to happen. This is especially necessary if you are planning to give birth in a hospital that you don't really care for but don't have any other choice. Usually doctors and nurses will respect a written document, especially if it is signed by the hospital administrator or your attorney—a step you may have to take if you want to keep the baby with you at all times and not have a fetal monitor in sight. Make your list simple yet clear, keep a copy with you, give one to your doctor, and send one to the maternity ward prior to your due date.

Remember the joy and the power. Labor is a comparatively short but intense time. You may feel suspended in the moment and caught in a dance that is being choreographed without your input. Keep in touch with your inner strength and the love you hold for your soon-to-be born child. Speak your wants and needs to those supporting you. Don't be afraid to ask for help. Stay in the present, not counting contractions past or contractions to come. Laugh. Cry. Feel. You are giving birth to your new self: mother. Reach down for your baby as it emerges; both you and your child need to continue the physical link you have had for so long. All at once, the labor of birth will be over and the labor of parenting begun.

To Birth Attendants

In a perfect world, there would be free universal health care, a midwife in every town, and a woman-centered birthing center at every hospital. In a perfect world, women would have choices about where and with whom to give birth. But until our politicians see fit to provide the money for these services and doctors see fit to give up their godlike place in our health care system, we will have to make do with what we have.

As I write this chapter, the newspaper headlines read "Woman Gives Birth Under Siege." This story refers to a laboring woman in Utah who was held hostage in a birthing center by a gunman angry about his wife's tubal ligation; he wanted to kill the doctor who performed the surgery. The doctor slipped out with several babies and left the woman, her partner, her women friends, and the nurse in attendance to deal with the gunman and to help birth the baby. The laboring woman held her baby in, on purpose, for four hours because she feared for the baby's life—a wonderful example of control under stress. I now suggest to you that women are giving birth under siege every day—taken prisoner by insensitive doctors and nurses, outdated hospital policies, and intrusive machines.

It is up to those of us who care to stop this siege. Here are my suggestions:

The family must stay together the entire time. The woman's chosen partner and friends have the right to be with her at all times (unless she says otherwise). If hospital personnel have a problem performing procedures in front of extra people, they should look at their reasons why—afraid of malpractice? afraid of not performing well? embarrassed?—and work on overcoming their fears. Likewise, the newborn should stay with the family at all times, unless the mother requests otherwise or the baby is *terribly* sick. The woman's partner should also be able to stay, and comfortable facilities should be available for him or her. The easiest way to accomplish all this is to have a "single room system" where there is no differentiation among labor, delivery, and postpartum areas—a woman and her family labor, give birth, and stay in the same room. It may cost the institution extra money to build or remodel such an area, but the postconstruction savings are enormous: less cleaning up, less equipment, happier staff, less infection, more consumers choosing such a special place.

Use technology appropriately. Look at policies and procedures that involve routine use of technology. Do all women really need a "twenty-minute strip" and blood and urine tests on admission? Perhaps these tests could be used for those who *really* need them rather than as a routine that does nothing more than protect against malpractice. If the "twenty-minute strip" is unavoidable, do it, then *get rid of the monitor.* Wheel it out of the room, get it out of sight. If it's in the room, it will be used. Better to monitor the baby—and the woman—with a well-trained nurse and a Doptone or fetoscope. Get babies out of isolettes unless they are really ill. If a baby simply needs to get warm, put him or her skin to skin with the mother under warm blankets. Never use a piece of equipment unless all noninterventionist solutions have been tried first. And remember, the technology itself may not be what is offensive to some birthing women, but the attitude with which it is used.

Provide the laboring woman with emotional and physical support instead of drugs. Something that midwives have known for centuries is just being recognized by the medical profession: that a woman has a shorter, easier labor if she has constant support from a trained woman—midwife, nurse, or doula (a trained lay woman who can be a labor assistant or mother's helper at home after the birth). When the going gets rough, suggest position changes, showers, or walks, and give her words of encouragement rather than "Would you like something for the pain, dear?" This question generally makes a woman feel bad and defeats her psychologically. The supportive presence of a doula, midwife, or nurse postpartum is also important, helping a woman and her partner with breast-feeding and newborn care.

Respect for the woman is paramount. The woman is at the center of the birth and should remain so. Everything that is done for her should be done with her permission after discussion and explanation. This goes for things as simple as taking her blood pressure and temperature or as complicated as surgery. The simple question "Would it be all right to change your bed/do a vaginal exam/check your urine?" with a reason why makes all the difference in the world. This respect extends to *all* women, not just educated, middle-class, white women. *All* women have the knowledge and power inside of them, and *all* deserve our respect and support. There is no need to cut a woman's perineum, for example, simply because she does not request "no episiotomy."

Do not do anything without a good reason. Explaining "because that's the way we've always done it" or "we're more comfortable with it that way" is not enough. You must have a *reason*. This was the most important thing I learned in nursing school. What is the good reason to have a multitude of sterile instruments opened for a birth when scissors, clamps, bulb syringe, towels, and placenta basin are enough? Other instruments can be available *if necessary.* This saves time and money, and helps the atmosphere to remain simple without taking on the air of high-tech. Why take a woman's vital signs at 7 A.M. when any time during the shift will do? Why limit breast-feeding to five minutes a side and only every four hours? Why have the woman's partner scrub and gown when she remains unscrubbed and ungowned? Think about everything you do—is there another way that is simpler, easier, more cost-effective, and more *respectful*?

The relationship among the birth attendants—nurses, doctors, and midwives—should be "horizontal." This means that each attendant should have an equally important role, that the doctor is not "better" than the midwife and the midwife is not "better" than the nurse. Each role is vitally important; each person is vitally important. One obvious way to develop this relationship is for all birth attendants to be on a first-name basis with each other. The feeling that comes with such respect is extraordinarily different from the traditional doctor/nurse hierarchy. Besides providing more satisfying working conditions for the birth attendants, this respectful atmosphere automatically spills over to and encompasses the birthing family.

Unfortunately, you may work in an institution where you are alone with your desires for change. There may be insensitive administrators or know-it-all doctors standing in your way. But one individual *can* make a difference. By using as many of my suggestions as possible within the realm of your choices, you may empower many women to find their inner strength and give birth. You may be stuck with continuous fetal monitoring, but you can do many things to help women change position and be more comfortable. You can ask their permission to do things, even if other staff members don't. You can respect the mother/infant unit by keeping them together as much as possible, by ignoring schedules and routines. Perhaps other staff members will begin to see the light—to understand that the woman and her family are more important than the staff; to understand that there are other, easier ways to do things; to understand that all labors and births are not meant to be alike, to fit into the same mold.

* * *

I dream that the day will come when *all* women will be respected for their choices, their strength, and their power. Birthing women have much to teach us if we can only let go of our preconceived notions about obstetrics. Birth is a mysterious time, full of heightened sensation and spontaneous actions. It is a time when women can truly be themselves and open up to the spirit of the new life inside. As birth attendants and pregnant women, we are all midwives, guiding the passage from one life to the next. Let us remain open to the possibilities, the differences, and the power. Together, let us have a safe and wonderful journey.

Index

About the Author

JANE DWINELL, R.N., a registered nurse for the past 15 years, has attended over 1,500 labors and 1,000 births at home, in the hospital, and at a birthing center. She has been published widely in prominent periodicals concerned with women's issues, health care, and country living skills.